ASPECTS OF ILLNESS

Cardiff Papers in Qualitative Research

About the Series

The Cardiff School of Social Sciences at Cardiff University is well known for the breadth and quality of its empirical research in various major areas of sociology and social policy. In particular, it enjoys an international reputation for research using qualitative methodology, including qualitative approaches to data collection and analysis.

This series publishes original sociological research that reflects the tradition of qualitative and ethnographic inquiry developed at Cardiff in recent years. The series includes monographs reporting on empirical research, collections of papers reporting on particular themes and other monographs or edited collections on methodological developments and issues.

Classics in Medical Sociology
An important new initiative featuring revised editions of influential titles in medical sociology.

Also available:
The Ceremonial Order of the Clinic
P.M. Strong and edited by Robert Dingwall

Aspects of Illness
Second edition

ROBERT DINGWALL
University of Nottingham

Ashgate

Aldershot • Burlington USA • Singapore • Sydney

Published by
Ashgate Publishing Limited
Gower House
Croft Road
Aldershot
Hants GU11 3HR
England

Ashgate Publishing Company
131 Main Street
Burlington, VT 05401-5600 USA

Ashgate website: http://www.ashgate.com

British Library Cataloguing in Publication Data
Dingwall, Robert
    Aspects of illness. - 2nd ed. - (Cardiff papers in
    qualitative research)
    1.Social medicine 2.Sick - Psychology
    I.Title
    306.4'61

Library of Congress Control Number: 2001093296

ISBN 0 7546 1670 3

Printed and bound in Great Britain by Antony Rowe |Ltd.,
Chippenham, Wiltshire.

Contents

Foreword to 2001 Edition

The justification for making this book available again reflects the extent to which two of the windmills at which it tilts continue to be with us and still need to be challenged. *Aspects* tried both to argue for the need for sociologists to be more critical of the positivist version of disease that was, and still largely is, hegemonic among our medical colleagues, and to insist that constructionist accounts cannot disregard the materiality of the human body and the disturbances to which its biology is subjected. Medical sociology remains pressed from each side.

The first chapter is directed mainly at the literature on illness behaviour and its attempt to specify social psychological models to explain why people act as they do in response to sickness. This line of work has continued into the currently fashionable Health Belief Model (Becker et al. 1972, Rosenstock et al.1988) and other social psychological models (Conner and Norman1996), to which much of the same critique can be applied. The arguments here are primarily methodological and reflect the early impact of ethnomethodological thinking on the group of medical sociologists then working in Aberdeen. In particular, they focus on the problem of the *post hoc* investigation of populations already classified by a medical diagnosis. Using Schutz's language, how can we derive 'in order to' motives from 'because of' motives, the processes involved in formulating and initiating actions from those involved in explaining and justifying them? The difficulties are compounded by the lack of evidence that the classification adopted by doctors for the purposes of specifying a diagnosis and an intervention has any original salience for the people presenting themselves for classification. Indeed, as Parsons (1951) understood and Freidson (1986,1994) has reiterated, we sometimes have to present ourselves to health professionals purely to have our self-classification affirmed for official purposes like access to social security or insurance benefits. Most of the time, though, we are brought to consult professionals because their licence (Hughes 1971), jurisdiction (Abbott 1988) or settlement (Abbott 2001) means that they know things that we do not.

The pragmatic achievements of this knowledge have, however, allowed its owners to assert an extensive mandate (Hughes 1971) over its application and development. In the present context, this is the 'pull of the policy audience' (Sarat and Silbey 1988) that has drawn a great deal of sociological effort into investigating the social correlates of medical classifications. This is a valuable enterprise but it should not be confused with the distinctive contribution that sociologists may be able to make to understanding how people come to decide that they are sick and what they then do about it. That enterprise is much less fashionable and receives less acknowledgment from the funders of health sciences research because it seems to be less practical or less keyed to their political agendas. In practice, however, as has been recognised increasingly over the last twenty years or so, it is a vital element in the development of effective interventions. Leaving aside those odd occasions on which we come more or less directly to the attention of health professionals - road accidents, collapses in the street, etc. - everything that the professionals have to deal with is filtered first through a process of self and lay assessment using whatever everyday knowledge is to hand. Moreover, which *Aspects* did not bring out at the time, what we do subsequent to professional intervention is also subject to the same filtration. If we want to change any of these processes, we still need a body of basic research on what lay people know, how they come to know it and how they use that knowledge. Without such work, many interventions to prevent ill-health, promote health or encourage concordance are simply a heartbreaking waste of time and money.

From the second chapter onwards, *Aspects* attempted to explore what a lay-centred study of illness might look like. Two points might be drawn out from this. The first is the implications of understanding illness as deviance. This was one of the great conceptual developments in medical sociology around 1970, although its foundation was really laid by Parsons (1951). This line of analysis has since gone into decline, for reasons that are not entirely clear. In part, though, it reflects the neglect of Parsons's attempt to think fundamentally about the nature of social organisation and the failure of medical sociologists to keep pace with the reappraisal of this, particularly by Camic (1987). The idea, that it makes a difference whether deviance is seen to be motivated or unmotivated, which Parsons elaborated in *The Social System*, is one of the most powerful tools that we have for exploring the differences in the control systems represented by medicine and by law. From this, we come to the second point, namely the value of seeing illness as some form of failure of everyday life. The argument for this is elaborated from what were then the unpublished lecture notes of Harvey Sacks (1995). Sacks showed that being ordinary was something that we had to work at. We had to know what it would take to 'be ordinary' and we had to be able to command the skills and resources, including our own bodies, to do this. The combination of Parsons and Sacks generated a view of illness as a failure of ordinariness that was not seen as intentional and therefore potentially triggered a range of micro and macro social response that were restorative and supportive, while still containing the deviance.

Throughout, however, there is an insistence on the *interaction* between human actors and their bodies that distinguishes *Aspects* from many later constructionist accounts. Schutz was particularly helpful here in his insistence on the phenomenon of 'imposed relevances'. Sometimes the material world is just there and we cannot do anything about it. At most we may have a modest degree of freedom to vary our constructions but we cannot define it as a pure act of will. Would you want to fly with a social constructionist airline pilot who thought that mountain ranges could be defined away? In the same fashion, the human body is subject to changes in its biological functions that are not matters of volition. A broken leg denies us some of the resources to do ordinariness, at least temporarily. An imperfectly repaired broken leg may deprive us of those resources permanently. The precise significance of these impairments will depend on both culture and technology. To what extent is mobility crucial to ordinariness in a given society - which may be quite different for hunter-gatherers or settled farmers? To what extent are compensating devices available - electric wheelchairs, golf buggies or whatever? An involuntary high fever is not the same as the voluntary ingestion of a psychoactive drug, even if each leads to an altered state of consciousness.

This acknowledgement of the *complementary* role of the sociology of the body and the biology of the body is also important in an appropriate respect for each. Parts of *Aspects* are under the spell of the nihilism about medicine provoked by Illich that has continued to compromise relations between social scientists and medical scientists over the last quarter of a century. It is easy to reach the conclusion that scientific knowledge is purely arbitrary from a study of its history and philosophy. The truths of one age turn out to be the errors of the next. Such a discovery, however, can easily lead us to overlook the movement that has taken place. This may not be as simple as the Whig histories of positivist science propose. Nevertheless, it is a movement and underlines the way in which the natural sciences are disciplined by the material world that they engage with. Of course, there are times when it is useful to stress the social dimensions of that knowledge and the discipline of materiality may be more or less present - theoretical physics is not the same as building bridges. Most of the time, though, the Second Law of Thermodynamics is not best thought of as a mere hypothesis.

The problem that *Aspects* did not solve, though, was that of a means of studying lay health knowledge. Some parts now look very strange, such as the espousal of Castaneda's work, which is now widely considered to have been fabricated (De Mille 1976, 1980). The main thrust, however, was on the potential of the formal methods used in what was variously known as componential analysis, ethnoscience or cognitive anthropology. This was a rather self-contained corner of American anthropology that never had much impact in Britain and did not achieve much more in the US, despite the distinguished efforts of Spradley (1979) and Agar (1973,1980, 1996). Agar (1982) argues that it was substantially absorbed by the broader field of cognitive science. In the process, it became less enamoured of the taxonomic approach described in *Aspects* and sought more flexible ways of representing the formal structures generative of culture, borrowing the idea of a *schema* from work in artificial intelligence. This is less a system of propositions than a set of instructions for the construction of propositions, a resource for performing cognitive tasks. The continuing search for a formal means of expressing the means of generating action that we might recognise as 'culture' has continued to set this work apart from the preference for empathic understanding that has since characterised a good deal of anthropological and anthropologically influenced ethnography. Nevertheless, its approach to trans-situational knowledge has attracted some ethnomethodologists and social constructionists, particularly in the workplace studies tradition. Their increasing suspicion of interview data (Dingwall 1997) would apply equally to formal elicitation. However, there is certainly a pragmatic argument, which would owe something to Wittgenstein's case against the idea of a private language, that some knowledge must be trans-situational for social interaction to be possible. Once conversation analysts conceded the idea of a turntaking *system* that would imply a knowledge of operating principles, if not of programming rules, carried between encounters (Sacks et al.1974) , the question might become one of how much knowledge rather than whether there was any at all. This was, for example, Goffman's argument, best expressed in 'Felicity's Condition' (Goffman 1983). The work of later cognitive anthropologists like Hutchins (1980) offers one example of how this might get done. The reissue of *Aspects* will be justified above all if a new generation of readers are encouraged to try to find their own solutions.

Acknowledgements for the 2001 Edition

This edition reproduces the text of the original although for copyright and production reasons the figures have been redrawn. Most of this work was done by Edward Dingwall, to whom I am most grateful. A few original typographical errors have been silently corrected and the bibliography revised to reflect the later publication of some of the cited materials. The book has also acquired an index thanks to Pamela Watson's help and the new Foreword has benefited from the comments of Anne Murcott. I would like to take the opportunity to reiterate my particular thanks to Mick Bloor for his encouragement with the original In this more scrupulous age a co-authorship credit would probably be due to him for the first chapter in recognition of his generosity in allowing me to make such free use of his M.Litt work on illness behaviour.

Acknowledgements

This book originated in a course element on the Senior Honours option in Medical Sociology at the University of Aberdeen in 1974-5. 1 have further developed the ideas in close association with Mick Bloor, to whom I am particularly indebted for permission to draw on unpublished material and for his thorough reading and constructive criticism of drafts of this work. Various parts of the book have also benefited from the suggestions of Janet Askham, Bill Cowie, Angela Jackson, Sally Macintyre, Judy Payne, Phyllis Stewart, Pamela Watson and Katherine Williams. While writing this I have been supported by funds from the Medical Research Council and the Social Work Services Group of the Scottish Education Department. I must also thank Elizabeth Connon for her sterling efforts on the typewriter and the patience and good humour with which she has coped with the numerous revisions of the manuscript. The responsibility for the final version embodied here is my own.

Robert Dingwall
Institute of Medical Sociology,
University of Aberdeen

Introduction

This book is concerned with the attempts made by sociologists (and, to a lesser extent, doctors) to account for patterns of social conduct that are observably associated with periods of illness. I shall make a number of critical observations on past approaches to this issue and propose a number of alternative lines of inquiry. In particular, I shall argue that medical sociologists have confused the proper realms of biological and sociological inquiry, and that it is this confusion that lies at the heart of the paucity of genuinely informative work in this field.

The origins of this confusion are not without interest in themselves. Traditionally, medical sociologists have tended to identify the *sociological* problem of why people act in certain ways during periods of illness with the *social* problem of why people do or do not make proper use of the 'official' medical services by whom medical sociologists have largely been funded. By 'official' medical services I mean those providers of medical care operating under the auspices of a State-granted monopoly of legitimate practice. Politicians and administrators have frequently been disturbed by the failure of those who are apparently in the greatest need to take up the services that are available. In an attempt to solve this problem, they have called upon medical sociologists. For their part, most medical sociologists have been ready and willing to be co-opted, welcoming the opportunity to demonstrate their own social concern.

The pragmatic basis of medical sociology is an important factor if we are to understand a number of the major features of this treatment of the orthodox topic of illness behaviour, from which this present inquiry begins. The problems of illness behaviour are located outside the medical services and the service-providers. Explanations are sought in terms of the characteristics of sick individuals rather than in terms of their interaction with institutions and their staff. In particular, the notion of illness itself is excluded from most investigations; it is taken directly from medical practitioners and treated as a resource for the study rather than being studied as a problem in its own right. This uncritical acceptance of the view of the social world expressed through medical services is associated with the central role of medicine as an agency of social control involved in the maintenance of our present social order. If research is to prove acceptable to those who control access to institutions and to research funds, then it must conform to a certain extent with their views of the social order.

What are the characteristics of these views of social order, these versions of social reality, and how are they legitimated? Here I follow Douglas's (1971) position. He argues that one of the key features of the thinking of agents of social control, among whom we may include those who police the development of knowledge through their power over access to research funds and research, is their assumption that their own culture, particularly its moral rules, is absolute. This official absolutism has six basic properties:

(i)   It is assumed that all normal, adequate persons interpret the social world in exactly the same way, so that the same meanings are assigned to social events by all competent members of the society.

(ii)   It is assumed that the assignation of meaning is completely unproblematic, so that everyone, in all situations, can know with certainty what is the correct or incorrect interpretation.

(iii)   Social meanings are thought to be external to individuals and therefore independent of volition, with an existence and meaning in their own right.

(iv)   Social meanings are thought to be necessary, so that the individual cannot avoid their impact or exercise any choice over whether or not to invoke them.

(v)   Social meanings are taken to be a necessary part of reality, deriving their authority from some extra-human source.

(vi)   Social meanings are viewed as timeless and eternal, so that their field of application and relevance is unbounded in time or space.

People who diverge from this model are treated as pathological, as instances of imperfect rationality and questionable competence as moral actors and fit members of society.

This identification of rationality with a particular moral viewpoint finds an echo in the work of Habermas. In his essay on 'Technology and Science as "Ideology"', he follows Marcuse in criticising the Weberian concept of rationalisation. Weber argued that rationalisation was a characteristic feature of modern society, representing the implementation of formal rationality in social action, based upon the application of scientific and technical criteria. Marcuse and Habermas contend that Weber has confused the extension of formal rationality with the implementation of a specific form of political domination legitimised by appeals to technology and science. This sort of rationality is concerned merely with:

...the correct choice among strategies, the appropriate application of technologies, and the efficient establishment of systems (with *presupposed* aims in *given* situations) [and] removes the total social framework of interests in which strategies are chosen, technologies applied, and systems established, from the scope of reflection and rational reconstruction. (Habermas, 1971, p. 82)

Habermas distinguishes two forms of rationalisation in his usage: rationalisation 'from below' and rationalisation 'from above'. The former describes the process of the supersession of traditional relationships in everyday life by systems of purposive-rational action - organisations of labour and trade, communication and transport systems, state bureaucracy, education, law, health services, the military and the family. The latter relates to the problem of legitimation as traditional mythological or religious world views lose their force. Habermas suggests that modern science plays a particularly crucial role in this, since it conspires to reduce political or moral problems to technical ones.

... propaganda can refer to the role of technology and science in order to explain and legitimate why in modern societies the process of democratic decision-making about practical problems loses its function and 'must' be replaced by plebiscitary decisions about alternative sets of leaders of administrative personnel ... it can also become a background ideology that penetrates into the consciousness of the depoliticised mass of the population where it can take on legitimating power. (Habermas, 1971, p. 105)

The favoured version of legitimation is what Schroyer (1971, p. 298) calls 'prescriptive scientism'. This neo-positivist view holds that knowledge is inherently neutral, that there is a unitary scientific method and that the standard of certainty and exactness in the physical sciences is the only explanatory model for scientific vague, and I think such a criticism is justified. Much of this present work could indeed be subsumed under such a formulation. I take it that Schroyer is getting at the attempt to restrict the application of this formula to a very narrow range of contexts, marked by an impersonal mode of expression, a particular form of logic and the adoption of quantification to achieve precision. In the present context, though, it is particularly important not to dismiss the achievements of scientism. In medical investigations, research under its auspices has conferred important benefits upon mankind. I am concerned to repudiate the view that only research that conforms to this paradigm is worth heeding.

It is against such a background that the activities of medical sociologists need to be set. In their researches they have, not unreasonably, kept one eye on their own social competence. The absolutist claims of service-providers have been largely unquestioned and excluded from the same attention that has been paid to service-recipients, actual or intended. Medical sociologists have offered explanations cast in terms of individual or collective pathology and styled after the injunctions of prescriptive scientism. Their inquiries have been directed by absolutist principles and have warranted those same principles. The first chapter of this book documents this charge by an examination of some of the more influential explanations of the social consequences of illness that medical sociologists have put forward. In that chapter I analyse representative selections from the body of literature on illness behaviour and on attempts to formulate accounts of illness within that tradition. This is followed in chapter 2 by an examination of previous attempts to break with this tradition and to develop accounts of illness as social action rather than as mere behaviour.

Chapter 3 is an attempt to formulate some more positive proposals. In this chapter I review a number of suggestions concerning more adequate conceptualisations of illness. In chapter 4 I seek to develop from them, an account of illness based on the study of everyday life in our own society. These suggestions are illustrated in chapter 5 by a reworking of empirical accounts of psychoactive drugs, poliomyelitis, myocardial infarction and childbirth. The book ends with a chapter that seeks to set out a methodological programme by which the questions raised in the book might be further investigated.

1 Illness Behaviour: The Failure of Positivism

To formulate any critique, we must start from a background of what is known or supposed. Accordingly, I shall begin this account by reviewing the explanations that medical sociologists have traditionally offered to account for the observable patterns of conduct, particularly in relation to official medical services, that are displayed by sick people. This is a topic that has conventionally been labelled 'illness behaviour'. Following Bloor (1970), I have organised the material into studies whose approach is based on the individual and those that approach the topic from the point of view of the collectivity. The former attempt to account for observed behaviour by reference to the personal characteristics of individuals; these may be socio-demographic indices or may be derived from some form of psychometric assessment. The latter seek to place individuals at the nexus of a balance of social forces and to account for their behaviour in terms of the forces that impinge. I have selected a number of classic examples of each of these tendencies for more detailed description and review. These are followed by a brief discussion of the immanent criticisms of the work from within the paradigm under which their authors are working. My central argument in this chapter, though, is that this paradigm is fundamentally inadequate and that our efforts should be directed towards replacing it rather than merely tinkering with it. The second part of the chapter is devoted to a more detailed exposition of the basic limitations of this approach, particularly when attempts have been made to examine the prior phenomenon of illness itself. In general, I hope to substantiate my initial charge that this approach is both absolutist and scientistic and that its consequent failure to confront social events on their own terms lies at the heart of its general defects.

Individualistic Models
(This section and the next draw heavily on unpublished work by Bloor, 1970.)

1 Rosenstock (1966)
Rosenstock's paper is an attempt to review and synthesise a number of earlier

1

reports on illness behaviour. He describes the reported characteristics of high and low service-users and criticises studies that have merely plotted correlations between socio-demographic factors and service-utilisation rates. This approach, he comments, fails to specify the causal connections between the two sets of variables. He proposes, instead, a model based upon the intervention of the personal characteristics of actors in the sequence of decisions that constitute illness behaviour. This model presents decisions to

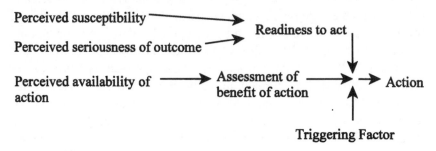

Figure 1.1 Rosenstock's model

seek medical attention as outcomes of the interaction of two variables. Firstly, there is the sufferer's psychological state of readiness to take action, which itself derives from his perception of his susceptibility to a condition and of the seriousness of the consequences of his having contracted that condition. Secondly, there is the extent to which the individual thinks that any particular course of action is likely to be beneficial in reducing the threat of the illness. This itself depends upon his views of the benefits of any given service and the possible barriers to its use. These two major variables require some cue for action to trigger them. Such cues Rosenstock sees as deriving from interpersonal events in a rather unspecified fashion. These three elements - readiness to act, assessment of benefit and triggering cue - are engaged in a balance of forces. A high level of readiness may need only a slight trigger to provoke action and vice versa.

The model in figure 1.1 was developed from comparisons between the studies, which are then cited as providing evidence for it. This introduces a certain circularity into attempts to justify its status, although, in fairness, Rosenstock does spell out in some detail what he would regard as relevant further research on the model depending upon reliable and valid quantification. A more crucial problem derives from the structure of the model. It uses a psychological variable - readiness to act - to explain why *some* action takes place, while the actor's perceptions explain *what* action takes place. The psychological variable, however, is treated as dependent on further variables relating to actors' perceptions, which are regarded as independent. In this respect Rosenstock is somewhat inconsistent, since he also argues that these perceptions are themselves socially generated. Any decision to treat them as independent must be arbitrary and considerably handicaps attempts to explain the social distribution of the psychological variable. Illness behaviour is seen to vary in association with the socio-demographic factors and this is taken to indicate variations in both the psychological and the social elements of the model. A more satisfactory way to account for this would seem to involve restoring the links between perception and culture, so that perception ceases to be an independent variable. In this case, Rosenstock's psychological interpolations seem redundant. How are we to recognise a 'state of readiness to act', apart from deducing it *post hoc* from some observed conduct? If we can recognise it only by this *post hoc* linking of consequent and supposed antecedent, how can it have any predictive status?

2a Mechanic (1962a, 1962b); Mechanic and Volkart (1961)
This model is based on Mechanic's research, with several student groups, into the relative influence of social stress and the social-psychological variable, 'readiness to adopt the sick role', on illness behaviour. In its structure, the consequent model is rather similar to Rosenstock's. One contingency, 'stress', explains why *some* action takes place, and another, 'inclination to adopt the sick role', explains *what* action takes place. Mechanic adopts a simple form of psychometric testing in order to measure these two factors and to determine their contribution to the observable conduct. In general, he argues, people under stress (defined as a state of affairs characterised by anxiety, discomfort, emotional tension and adjustment) have a repertoire of coping responses. One of these is the adoption of the sick role, as formulated by Parsons (1951). Variations in the use of medical services can be put down to variations in individual propensity to experience stress and to adapt to it by assuming the sick role. The model (see figure 1.2) is further elaborated by the introduction of another variable, 'perceived symptomatology'. People with a low inclination to adopt the sick role would be likely to seek treatment only if they experienced particularly unusual or severe symptoms.

But Mechanic, too, is confronted by the problem of accounting for the systematic social distribution of illness behaviour. He attempts to do this by depicting coping responses as learned behaviour. If this is the case, then

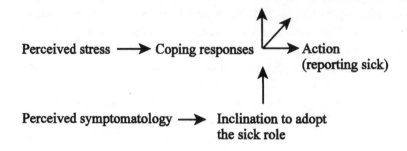

Figure 1.2 Mechanic's model

presumably the perceptual aspects of the model must also be learned. As with Rosenstock, these modifications pull us away from the individualism of the model towards a greater stress on social and cultural elements. Mechanic confines himself to showing associations between an inclination to adopt the sick role and various socio-demographic factors, but he cannot, within this model, show how such an association arises. The associations do not have any causal import but merely describe more or less constant conjunctions. The links between the conjoined events remain to be described. In this case, such a task could be accomplished only by appeals to commonsense, by what we all take to be true about certain kinds of people, rather than by empirical investigation.

One can also add that Mechanic omits any discussion of the availability of medical services (partly because his data are drawn from a campus with a readily available health service) and of the availability of the option of adopting the sick role. This, too, may reflect the population from which the model is drawn, who may have relatively fewer economic or social obligations to restrict the availability of this option. One may also note the general problems of validity in psychometric investigation. A detailed consideration of this issue is beyond the scope of the present discussion but is well documented elsewhere (Cicourel, 1964, 1974; Friedman, 1967; Phillips, 1973).

2b Mechanic (1968)

This version is not strictly an individualistic one, but it is convenient to consider it here. In his textbook on medical sociology, Mechanic seems to abandon his earlier model, indeed to abandon any attempt at model-building, in favour of merely listing ten heterogeneous variables that other studies have shown are associated with illness behaviour. Each variable is manifested in both self- and other-defined forms. The variables are:

(i)   the visibility, recognisability or perceptual salience of deviant signs and symptoms;

(ii) the extent to which the symptoms are perceived as serious;

(iii) the extent to which symptoms disrupt family, work and social activities;

(iv) the frequency of the appearance of deviant signs or symptoms, their persistence or their frequency of occurrence;

(v)   the tolerance threshold of others;

(vi) the available information, knowledge and culture assumptions and understandings of the sufferer;

(vii) basic psychological needs which lead to autistic psychological processes (i.e. perceptual processes that distort reality);

(viii) the needs that compete for attention with response to the illness;

(ix) the competing interpretations that can possibly be assigned to recognised symptoms;

(x)   the cultural, social and economic availability of treatment resources.

Apart from the convenience of summarising a large body of previous work and indicating the general issues that are likely to be involved in any attempt to account for illness behaviour, this inventory does not help us very much. In some ways, it may even hinder our understanding by implying a model based simply on these ten factors, with each item reified into an independent variable and the overlaps and interrelations left unexamined. Mechanic's review also tends to treat all the studies cited as equally valid and to disregard their methodological variety.

3 Kosa et al. (1966), Kosa and Robertson (1969)

Kosa's model is sketched out in the 1966 paper which reports on a series of studies of the distribution of illness episodes based on industrial absentee records and on self-reporting of symptoms by means of family health diaries. It is elaborated in a more general review of the field in the later paper. Illness episodes are broken down into four parts:

    (i)   the assessment of a disturbance in, or of a threat to, the usual functioning of physiological-psychological health;

    (ii)   the arousal of anxiety by such an incident;

    (iii) the application of one's general medical knowledge to the given disturbance;

    (iv) the performance of manipulative actions for removing the anxiety and the disturbance.

In this model, like the others, one contingency, 'anxiety', explains why some action takes place, while another, 'the application of general medical knowledge', explains what action took place. Anxiety plays an important role in this account. There are two types of anxiety involved here: firstly, specific anxiety about any threat to one's security and physical and psychological well-being, aggravated in the case of sickness by the ultimate anxiety of death; and secondly, general or floating anxiety present in the psychological mechanism of any person, which may be released and focussed on the particular case in hand. This anxiety is structured by the application of individual and collective general medical knowledge, which is developed and transmitted within particular cultural settings. Variations in the social distribution of this knowledge can lead to instances of culture clash between clients and professionals and account for the low rates of take-up of official services by some groups of potential patients. The application of this knowledge leads to a variety of manipulative actions directed at satisfying the basic psychological need (relieving anxiety) by changing the objective situation (the disturbance of health). Throughout, Kosa emphasises the affectual rather than the cognitive dimensions of action.

This emphasis on the affectual does tend to inhibit the explanatory value of Kosa's position. Although it is a salutary reminder that illness is an emotional matter for most sufferers, the view that important elements of the model are non-rational does rather place them beyond the possibility of empirical study, except in the speculative manner of psychoanalysis. Beyond this, Kosa is also rather vague about the relationships between the elements of his model. It is difficult to see how perception of a disturbance in normal functioning can be separated from general medical knowledge, which presumably provides for the identification of states of being as either disturbances or normal functioning. Similar problems arise with the distinction between applying medical knowledge and performing manipulative actions, particularly if we accept Schutz's (1964) analysis of recipe knowledge, which suggests that the identification of typical problems and the initiation of remedial action are not clearly separable in commonsense thinking. It is also unclear how Kosa's model relates to the experiences of a patient within an official medical system as opposed to experiences in the lay community. A more satisfactory analysis would need to account for various forms of professional consultation and intervention.

Collectivity-orientated Models

1 Zola (1965, 1966)

Zola's analysis is based on a series of studies which investigated the illness behaviour of different ethnic groups in the Boston area. In his view, 'objective' symptomatology was part of the normal condition of most people most of the time. The decision to take action or seek help on any particular occasion did not seem to be related in any systematic fashion to the severity of the symptoms. For him, the problem had to be seen as one of explaining the decision to seek medical aid at a particular point in time. He attributed this to a break in the sufferer's ability to accept his normal symptomatology, provoked by some trigger. Five varieties of triggers were identified:

    (i)   the occurrence of an interpersonal crisis;

    (ii)   perceived interference with social or personal relations;

    (iii)   the sanctioning of the sufferer's condition by others;

    (iv)   perceived interference with vocational or physical activity;

    (v)   a sudden change in the normal symptomatology.

In any given case, Zola found that the effective trigger was related to the ethnicity and educational level of his respondents. The first and second were commonest among Italians, the third among Irish and the fourth and fifth among Anglo-Saxons. Zola attributed this to variations in culturally transmitted ways of responding to crises. These cultural influences on the perception, presentation and management of illness account for variations in the presentation of disorders to official medical agencies.

This study presents certain analytical and methodological problems. Firstly, it is not immediately apparent that the first four triggers are as independent as Zola suggests. If they overlap substantially the supposed ethnic correlations may result more from the commonsense imputations involved in the researcher's coding decisions on what is to count as an example of a trigger than from the events themselves. These decisions and their basic data may also be influenced by ethnic differences in the interviews from which the material was collected. Interview data are the product of a social encounter, and we need to analyse these encounters in the same way as any other social encounter before we can determine the status of reports based on them. The claims that Zola (1966, p. 625) makes on the basis of quotations from two interviews with Irish and Italian respondents, for example, cannot be accepted unless we know more about how the respondents saw the interviewer - the alleged ethnic differences in types of response may simply reflect ethnic differences in interview behaviour.

Secondly, Zola's work is based solely on people who had already presented themselves at official medical services, so that his explanations of patient presentation cannot be checked against the behaviour of non-presenters.

Thirdly, there is no attempt to specify the suggested links between behaviour and cultural milieux. Cultures, classes, occupations, families or whatever do not cause behaviour as a blow on the knee causes a reflex jerk.

Finally, Zola does not allow for the degree to which a patient's experience of illness may be influenced by interaction with hospital staff. If hospital staff share Zola's commonsense assumptions about the behaviour of ethnic groups, they may well act in ways that help to generate the behaviour they anticipate. These in turn are a factor in the accounts that patients are likely to give of their illness experience.

2 Suchman (1964, 1965); Rosenblatt and Suchman (1965)

Suchman's analysis is based on data collected in a survey of the medical contacts of a probability sample taken from an ethnically and socially heterogeneous district of New York. Suchman tried to account for the observable variations in the take-up rates of official medical services in terms of the organisation of an individual's social relationships and his orientations towards medical care. Cohesive community groups may be more independent of official medical care systems, since the individual is supported in deviant beliefs.

Their underutilization of modern medical facilities and their lack of co-operation in community health programs may be simply one more expression of their general estrangement from the mainstream of middle-class American society. In this respect 'medical' disorganization among these groups becomes another form of social disorganization. (Suchman, 1964, p. 331)

This line of argument bears some resemblance to Parkin's (1967) account of Labour voting as social deviance sustainable only in relatively homogeneous working-class areas which can offer a systematic alternative to the dominant conservative national culture. Parkin does not however share Suchman's absolutist view of this alternative system as pathological, a symptom of social disorganisation. We shall return to this particular issue, but it is necessary to recognise the difference between pluralist and absolutist views of cultural diversity.

We can represent Suchman's thesis in a diagrammatic form (Figure 1.3).

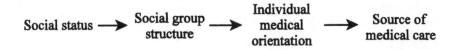

Figure 1.3 Suchman's original model

'Social status' describes the individual's class position and 'social group structure' seems to refer to the nature of the social networks in which he participates. Suchman and his team interviewed in more depth a randomly selected group of the original sample. From these data they sought to assign scores to their respondents on various scales reflecting the dimensions of the model particularly group structure and medical orientation. Unfortunately, however, these data failed to support this straightforward model and Suchman was obliged to revise it (Figure 1.4).

Bloor (1970, p. 29) argues that this still fails to reflect the data obtained in the study. A direct relationship is retained between social group structure and medical care, for example, although the study failed to provide empirical evidence of this. The model also proposes a curiously direct relationship between socio-demographic factors (ethnicity and socioeconomic status) and medical orientation. How can these factors be said to cause a particular way of viewing the social world? Might it not be more satisfactory to suppose that they are mediated through the same interpretive processes that give rise to orientations to medical intervention? Suchman also makes the curious assumption that cohesive social groups are uniquely lower-class phenomena and, by definition, incompatible with a favourable orientation towards official medical services. Kadushin's (1966) work on recruitment to psychotherapy among the New York intelligentsia clearly demonstrates that this view is incorrect.

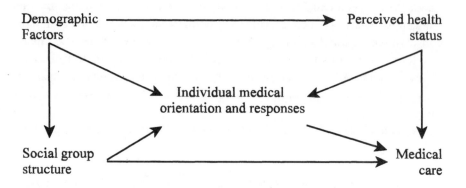

Figure 1.4 Suchman's revised model

Suchman's model of the decision to seek medical help is embedded in an account of the processes of a pre-patient career, identifying three stages: 'symptom experience', 'assumption of the sick role' and 'medical care contact'. At each stage new problems confront the sick individual and new information is fed into the model to generate new or revised decisions. However, the status of these career stages and the links between them remain rather elusive. I suspect that this partly reflects the general difficulties inherent in the search for a single meta-career that can account for all contingencies and subsume all particular careers. Such meta-careers have to be formulated at a level of abstraction that divorces them from any clear empirical reference. They therefore tend to become sociological legislations of what social reality ought to look like, rather than second-order redescriptions of events in terms that can, in principle, be translated into the accounts that individuals themselves use to produce and interpret those events. Given this divorce between the version of social order produced by sociologists and the version produced by the people they have studied, it is not surprising that sociologists' accounts have a somewhat limited use.

Immanent Criticism

Before criticising the basic paradigm that has traditionally been employed in this area, I want to examine the problems that have been identified within the prevailing theoretical and methodological tendencies by people working under the auspices of those tendencies. One of the fullest analyses is that of McKinlay (1972), and this section follows his organisation of material. Although his review is more narrowly confined to utilisation behaviour, this is not clearly separable from the general issue of illness behaviour and most of his comments are equally applicable to either. He laments the general lack of consistency, co-ordination and coherence in empirical work, and of a sound theoretical basis for research in the area. He identifies seven specific problems.

1 Sources of data
Most research into the use of official medical services is derived from one of three sources: doctors' records; hospital, clinic or insurance records; or sample surveys. Doctors' records present difficulties in gaining access to them and extracting usable information from them. Hospitals, clinics and insurance companies tend to keep their records in a form that facilitates central reporting and makes them more useful for research, although they are more useful for planners and administrators concerned with organising and evaluating specific services than for those involved in fundamental research. McKinlay does not elaborate on this, but clearly Garfinkel's (1967, pp. 186-207) observations on record-keeping are important here. He notes that organisational records are contractual rather than actuarial. They are not literal descriptions of events, but accounts organised in such a way that the organisation's members can, if necessary, point to them to defend their conduct as reasonable. They may provide useful information for people working within the conceptions about the organisation's tasks and their performance current in the organisation, but they have only a limited use for anyone working independently.

The other source of data noted by McKinlay is the sample survey. This involves asking people not selected by the use of official services about their symptoms and behaviour. There are, however, known tendencies towards under-reporting owing to the fallibility of memories, the stigma attached to some conditions, a reluctance to communicate with an interviewer of the opposite sex and a variety of other situational factors. Many of these studies fail to distinguish between true non-users and those classified as non-users merely because there is no record of medical consultation. Phillips (1972) also notes how the social nature of interviews can bias responses. In an interview the respondent is likely to want to present himself as a 'good subject'. The answers given are those which the respondent defines as 'answers-to-the-interviewer's questions', possibly leading to the suppression of material that the respondent believes to be trivial and insignificant, or liable to give the interviewer a poor opinion of him.

2 Sampling problems

Two issues arise here - the definition of the population to be sampled, and the most appropriate way of using survey material to study a social process like illness behaviour and the consequent use of services. Most research in this area has concentrated on fairly limited populations, drawn either from single cities or areas or, even more specifically, from clients of a single service. Subsequent findings may, then, be of very limited significance and may conceal the intervention of class or regional factors. In the United Kingdom, it cannot be lightly assumed, for example, that what is true for London is equally true for Scotland, Wales or even the rest of England. Similarly, a disturbingly large proportion of published American work seems to be drawn from public health facilities in the North-East. The findings *may* hold true for private health care and for other regions, but this cannot be taken for granted. In spite of the practical difficulties involved, national data of some kind seem to be needed if the limitations of local investigations are to be reliably determined.

The second set of difficulties relates to the problems involved in trying to study social processes by means of social surveys. Two options are suggested: one might take a cross-section of the population at some fixed point in time, including people at a variety of stages of illness; or one might take a panel that could be studied over time. The first method is considerably easier, since respondents have to be interviewed only on a single occasion and do not have to he traced and persuaded to co-operate on several occasions. On the other hand, it does present problems of deducing antecedents from consequents. The investigator has to assume that his respondents' answers fall into certain patterns and that the career stages described by some members of the sample can be retrospectively linked to career stages reported by other members of the sample. The prospective nature of panel studies reduces this problem, if all panel members start at the same point. On the other hand, panel members' behaviour may be altered by their participation in the research.

3 Quantity versus quality

There has been a tendency merely to appraise services in terms of the quantity of care that has been given, without regard to its quality. 'Quality' can involve both the quality of the medical treatment itself and the subjective responses of clients to the social aspects of the service.

4 Retrospectivity

Studies have usually been based on people who have already received a service. This clearly presents problems in relation to the accurate recall of past events. This is not merely a question, as McKinlay implies, of the fallibility of memory, but also a question of the extent to which any account of past events is reconstructed to suit present contingencies. Disentangling causality, as McKinlay notes, presents a genuine problem. If statements of belief or attitude are collected after observed behaviour, we can say either that the beliefs caused the behaviour or that the behaviour caused the belief.

5 The decision-making process

The means whereby individuals approach a service have been relatively neglected. All that is known is that there are correlations between crude socio-demographic indices and specific behaviour. McKinlay doubts whether further research into this aspect is really justifiable and argues for studies of the social processes that are involved in producing these demonstrable associations.

6 Individualism

With a few exceptions, research has concentrated on the specific psychological characteristics of clients to explain the failure of potential clients to use services. This has in part been superseded by ideas of the 'culture of poverty' or, in Britain, 'transmitted deprivation'. These share a common strategy of 'blaming the victim', attributing the failings of the poor to their alleged inadequacies, rather than considering the structural availability and relevance of services.

7 Forms of service

Researchers have tended to be rather uncritical about the organisations that offer services. They have tended to assume both that individuals have similar relationships with all services they encounter, and that any given form of service is equally appropriate for all potential users.

McKinlay's general prescription for these ills involves methodological, empirical and theoretical issues. Firstly, he urges more small-scale inductive studies, more attention to replication and prospective research and more detailed sociodemographic work. Secondly, he puts forward a case for greater attention to the social context of illness behaviour, using the concept of 'social network'. It is also important to consider help seeking in illness as a process and to develop descriptions of help-seeking careers. Finally, McKinlay calls for greater attention to the client-agency interface and the negotiation of patterns of conduct. We should probably add to this list the question of the social context of service availability. There are likely to be important differences in use where services are under political pressure to restrict availability.

The Failure of Positivism

I do not believe that McKinlay's proposals offer us any genuine advance. They remain cast in the mould of the traditional paradigm in this area, a paradigm with which, I argue, we must break if we are to develop a *sociology* of illness and illness behaviour. Throughout this account, I have tended to imply the nature of that paradigm. It is now time to make it explicit.

Positivism is a much-abused word in contemporary sociology. Its usage has departed considerably from that current in philosophy, to the confusion of many people. In this section I am using it in the strictly sociological sense, which might be better served by the term 'scientism' (Schroyer, 1971, p. 298). Giddens (1974, pp. 3-4) and Schroyer both present this perspective as involving three basic suppositions.

(i)   The methodological procedures of natural science may be directly adopted by sociology so that scientific method is not merely unitary but also homogeneous between all fields of human inquiry. Social conduct may be treated as an object in the same way as natural objects, and the phenomena of subjectivity, volition and will present no particular problems.

(ii) The goal of the social analyst is to formulate laws or law-like statements akin to those of the natural sciences and copying their standards of certainty and exactness.

(iii)   Sociology, and knowledge in general, has a purely technical character and is inherently neutral with respect to values or practical implications.

Most research on illness and its consequences shares these features, which have been deeply entrenched in English-speaking sociology since the Second World War. They have contributed greatly to the acceptability of medical sociology in the United States, in medical circles where research operates under similar intellectual assumptions. In Britain the situation has been slightly different, since medical sociology has had to compete with an entrenched medical specialty of social medicine. Social medicine research has also, naturally enough, followed a scientistic model, and British sociologists' endeavours have for the most part represented a pale shadowing. It is clearly easier to gain access to a medical community by accepting its model of inquiry and following its prescriptions of appropriate methods, a search for predictive statements and a purely technical mode of inquiry. However, one can argue that the consequence has been a gross distortion of sociological investigation, which has done a disservice to both sociology and medicine.

Let us first take up the issue of the scientific status of social inquiry. Here, I suggest, the form of the scientific method has been mistaken for its content. This has consequences both for the conduct of research and for the status of the subject of that research. Scientistic sociology is deeply concerned with the precise measurement and quantification of phenomena and it is argued that the social sciences can develop only through mathematisation. Yet why have the natural sciences adopted quantification? To achieve the precise description of phenomena. These phenomena are objects that merely behave, since, so far as we know, they lack language and are therefore incapable of intentional action. This means that some community of scientists can erect a system for assigning numbers to properties of phenomena by common consensus. Everybody can come to agree about what it means to say that an event happens x times in y minutes or that factor A is n times greater than factor B. And of course, since the phenomena are not intentional actors and cannot answer back, the natural scientist can describe the behaviour of the objects of his study without the arbitrary nature of the correspondence between his descriptions and the events under study being a practical problem.

We can take as an example the addition of some substance to a sample of blood to examine its effects on white cells. Now it is relatively easy to agree on how to count those cells before and after the addition of this substance, to be able to say that there are x cells per mm^3 or whatever. Scientists can agree on what is to stand as an instance of one unit of the phenomenon being investigated. If we add some chemical and find that the white cell count is depressed, then we naturally infer that it is the action of that chemical that has caused this reduction. We do not get the white cells turning round and arguing that it is the physical act of adding the chemical, rather than the chemical itself, that is really important. It is quite irrelevant that the account we give of observable events is not a literal description of those events, but merely a version of them that agrees with the consensus among scientists about how they are to be described. This does not prevent us from deriving important practical benefits from the partial reports of natural scientists. It would clearly be absurd to argue that such a way of doing natural science should be completely abandoned.

But if we want to find out how patients react when they are ill, the situation is rather different. We can describe this in biological terms - that in the presence of such and such a foreign organism certain physical changes took place - and, at one level, this is a complete explanation. But if we want to move from the biological sphere to the behavioural sphere, the situation changes. We can say that the patient exhibits certain behavioural signs, like the tremors of Parkinson's Disease, that are beyond his voluntary control. We can also say that the patient reports certain symptoms or manifests disturbances of voluntary conduct. Ignoring for the moment the very real problem of discriminating between voluntary and involuntary behaviour, we are faced with the difficulty of establishing equivalence classes for conduct. It is easy for the natural scientist to recognise that two instances of some phenomenon are the same. He can add substance S_1 to substance S_2 and get reaction R, and recognise that each time he repeats the procedure the events will belong to the same class. This possibility is not open to the social scientist. Equivalence classes can be established only if we make some reference to the intentions of the individual in the situation he is in. If we take the simple matter of raising an arm, it is absurd to argue that there is a social equivalence between all occasions of arm-raising. We need to know about both the intention and the situation. If a child raises his hand in a classroom there are a number of possible interpretations: he may wish to leave the room; he may wish to question the teacher; he may have cramp in his elbow and want to stretch his arm. We can decide between these only by asking him what he meant. But if we ask him what he meant his reply depends upon his reading of the situation. The child may be reluctant to admit to the class teacher that he had a 'trivial' reason for raising his arm, like suffering from cramp, and proffer a 'serious' one, like a need to visit the lavatory. To a friendly observer he may concede that he was suffering from cramp. So even reports of intentions are intentional acts. Indeed, all speech is necessarily intentional.

If we think it worth while we can use scientistic methods to describe human *behaviour*. We can count the number of times we see children raising their arm in the classroom. But we must agree what it means to raise an arm. Is it to shoulder height or beyond? Does the arm have to be fully extended? Does it have to be vertical, oblique or horizontal? We can count the number of times children tell us they raised their arm because they had cramp, because they wanted to ask a question or because they wanted to leave the room and casually ignore the problem of equivalence between these answers. We can find associations between arm-raising for particular reasons and the size of classroom, time of day, distance from lavatories, age and sex of teacher or whatever. But all this gives us is a partial description that bears no known relation to the events it purports to describe, since it is entirely produced by the classification of the researcher. If we want to move beyond this to the study of human *action,* we must adopt a theory and method that take account of the intentions of the actors in their proper context. I shall return to this point, but I want to emphasise that I do not want to discredit the appeal for precise observation and description, merely the claim that this can be achieved only by quantification. The unity of the scientific method does not lie in a homogeneity of technique or procedural logic, but in what Schutz has called the 'scientific attitude', the cast of mind in which inquiry is undertaken.

I have already anticipated the argument on law-like statements. Basically, I argue that if human conduct is seen as intentional action, the possibility of formulating laws disappears. In my reading, intentionality necessarily involves some element of will. While the exercise of that will may be restricted by the elements present in any given situation, the very availability of elements is itself shaped by the individual's purposes, the exercise of his will. Let us suppose we are trapped by fire in our bedroom. Our intention is to escape. The ideal may be to climb down a ladder, but, like most bedrooms, ours does not have a ladder in it. Our possible actions are restricted by the unavailability of a ladder. On the other hand we have read novels where the hero escapes down a rope of knotted sheets. So the sheets on the bed suddenly become available in a new light. At other times our intentions have made them available as something to sleep between. Now they are a potential means of escape. If we had not read the relevant novels, or if there had been no fire, they might have remained unavailable for such action. We can make a link between the fire and the action of stripping the bed and knotting sheets together only by some reference to the processes whereby we recognised the fire, made sense of its occurrence and formulated possible responses.

In the social sciences one cannot make statements of the typical form of a scientific law, 'if X, then Y'. We can merely offer *post hoc* accounts, 'X, because of Y', or prophecies, 'if X, then probably Y', if X is seen in some particular way, Z_1, or Y_2 ... if... Z_2 or Y_n ... if Z_n. The sociologist may be able to make informed suggestions about what is likely to happen or why things happened as they did, but he cannot say what *will* happen. The attempts of social behaviourists to produce laws founder on their inability to specify causal links between events, since they exclude individuals' purposes from their investigations. They merely produce descriptions of constant conjunctions.

Finally, we must note the prevailing assumption of the technical character of research. Here again, I suggest, there is some confusion. While the methods of social inquiry may be neutral with respect to values, the context in which they are used is not. Theories, whether social or scientific, are the ways in which we bring order into the world. They allow us to make sense of what we see before us. These theories are the ways in which we demonstrate our own rationality, so that they inevitably reflect our own circumstances. We can show that we are a competent doctor or a competent sociologist by demonstrating our ability to make reference to the theories that are current among doctors or sociologists at the present time. And, of course, theories about the world also include methods for getting to know that world. So while methods themselves may be neutral, their use inevitably comes within the context of a theory and hence within the context of a set of social interests and moral choices. This may not have much practical importance for the natural scientist, for whom the morally based nature of his theorising is seldom a problem; but it does matter for the student of social life, since the plausibility of his reports cannot be adequately assessed unless we understand the circumstances of their development. Sociology necessarily reflects more critically on its own practice than do most natural sciences. This derives from its growing recognition of the plural nature of knowledge and of social order.

In this context it is essential to underline the differences between pluralist and absolutist versions of knowledge. Prescriptive scientism is an absolutist version which holds that it has a unique access to truth. This is a very seductive claim to elitist researchers. It allows us to believe that our view of the world is necessarily and exclusively true. The dogmatist can present his particular construction of reality as objectively and uniquely real. The dogma may be of the Right or the Left, of Catholic or Protestant, of White supremacy or Black supremacy. It is no less dogma, no less elitist, no less absolutist. Absolutism discredits any and all alternatives. Against this, pluralism recognises the infinite variety of views that may be adopted and their equal integrity. All accounts of the world are seen as having an equal epistemological status, although their practical efficacy may vary. Western science has traditionally taken an absolutist view of itself. It presents itself as a collection of truths. Science has not felt it necessary to examine the conditions of its existence. It merely investigates a world that is given to it. Traditionally, sociology has tended to follow a similar model. Recent years, however, have seen the development of pluralist alternatives in ethnoscience and ethnosociology. The terms are derived from the Greek *ethnos,* a people. What we are talking about is the study of the science of peoples, the modes of knowledge and explanation which members of a society themselves bring to make sense of the social and natural world. Magic, religion, politics, science, sociology can all be seen as folk systems for understanding the world. They can all be taken equally seriously.

Health Beliefs

It is this failure to take lay beliefs seriously that characterises most traditional research in medical sociology. The work on illness behaviour displays all the characteristics of both absolutism and scientism. It relies almost exclusively on various forms of statistical investigation into features of lower-class subjects' worlds that the investigator thinks ought to be important. The problem is located in the individual or social pathology of the subjects, whose behaviour is treated as odd and irrational by the unexamined standards of the researchers. This should not be read as an attack on the integrity of these workers. One of the marked features of this field has been the humane and pragmatic concern of its investigators. For the most part, these are people who genuinely want to improve the lot of those who are poor, black or otherwise excluded from a share of power in their own society. But it is this very practical element that has led to the relative neglect of fundamental theoretical issues. All the time people have wanted to *do* something, to change the world before they have understood it. Naturally, then, they adopted the most influential models of theory and method that were available to them. In part this reflected the prestige of scientism among the governing classes. Research that was to persuade them had to be in a form that they would find plausible. In part it reflected the authors' own liberalism, with its belief that the American intelligentsia represented the furthest advance of Western civilisation. Both of these assumptions have since been severely shaken by the ecological movement and by the Vietnam War. Even to write neutrally about them can sound satirical or patronising. The absolutist thought of these investigators was different in content from the absolutism of business or the military, but its form was the same and it blinded its adherents just as much to the integrity of the groups under study.

By way of drawing the themes of this chapter together, I want to return to a more detailed and explicitly critical examination of some research into the fundamental issue of illness as a social phenomenon, in order to demonstrate how this paradigm is ultimately incapable of coping with any of the basic issues in the explanation of social action.

Kirscht *et al.* (1966) report on an American national survey of health beliefs in relation to cancer, tuberculosis, tooth decay and gum disease. They aimed to investigate perceptions of the severity of, and likely susceptibility to, these conditions and the potential benefits of preventive action and early diagnosis. Questionnaires were administered to 1,493 adults in seventy geographical areas in the United States. The authors state that the conditions were selected 'to provide a range of objective clinical severity and to represent problems of continued and increasing concern to public health'. Immediately we have an explicit absolutist commitment. Firstly, the diseases selected and named in the questionnaire are scientific medicine's diseases. We do not know what place they fill, if any, in the respondents' theories about illness. Are these diseases that they would recognise and respond to in identical terms to those used by the clinician? If we do not know this, how can we argue that the respondents' replies have any significance, beyond that of a desire to play their part in the interview? Secondly, the conditions are of a range of 'objective' severity. By what standards? This arrogation of objectivity is a common feature of absolutism. Objective criteria of severity exist only within a theoretical context and, as we have seen, theories are socially situated phenomena. Thirdly, we have the expressed concern with problems of public health. Who are the public? Obviously cancer, tuberculosis and so on are unpleasant, even fatal, but any talk of problems of public health involves an absolutist assertion of a moral claim. It is a claim that some group has the right to define healthy and unhealthy living standards, which it wishes to enforce as true for the whole society. Now this may indeed be of practical benefit to all parties. This author, for instance, would like to see tobacco smoking outlawed. It would improve his health and that of many other people. But let us not fool ourselves into thinking that this is not a moral assertion about private and public welfare and not an absolutist claim.

The methods of the study are thoroughgoing scientism. Let us take as an example the attempt to measure the threat involved in the various conditions. This has two elements: firstly, the use of a five-category Likert scale (of the type: I am very worried, worried, indifferent, unconcerned, very unconcerned) about each condition; secondly, the use of emotionally worded statements about each condition with which respondents were asked to agree or disagree. These both run up against the equivalence problem. How are we to know whether the respondents interpreted these in the way they were intended to when the questionnaire was devised? How are we to know whether each respondent's answers are equivalent to every other respondent's answers? Through such methods we arrive at a distribution of numbers. The researcher is then faced with the problem of finding some meaning in them. In this study, the conscientiousness of the investigators allows us to see the difficulty of this task. For example, in asking about the perceived threat of conditions, they ask this in relation both to the respondent and to 'people in general'. This was in order to investigate a quasi-psychoanalytic hypothesis that people who feel threatened are likely to engage in either projection or denial. Unfortunately they cannot tell which, since there is no way of knowing, in their terms, whether the 'true' distribution of beliefs is represented by the responses about oneself or the responses concerning others. If it is the former then we are seeing projection, in the greater perceived vulnerability of others; if the latter, we are seeing denial. Later in the paper beliefs are associated with socio-demographic variables such as age, sex, education and income. Here again we can see an attempt to fill in an explanation: 'Vulnerability to disease and helplessness in the face of disease tend to be associated with lower social status, possibly reflecting reduced ability and resources to cope with the environment.' The authors are impeccably cautious at this point, but their basic operation still involves drawing on some kind of commonsense notion of what 'lower-class' people are like to bridge the explanatory gap between their questionnaire responses and their social inventory of respondents.

This is not to say that none of the studies starts out from lay conceptions of illness. Apple (1960) and Baumann (1961), for example, both begin with lay concerns. Apple notes:

There has been little investigation of whether a layman who decides he is ill has based this conclusion, at least in part, on factors which a doctor would not consider to be untrue or imaginary but which rather are irrelevant to a professional judgement about the state of his health. Hence it seems important to find out the conditions under which the layman thinks of himself, or others, as being ill. (Apple, 1960, p. 219)

She presented a sample of sixty people aged between twenty and sixty years of age and controlled for sex and class, with eight fictitious descriptions of illness episodes. These were written to combine three elements that were thought to be relevant to lay definitions: interference with usual activities; the time that had elapsed since onset; and degree of ambiguity. She does not account for the origin of these ideas. Are these again merely commonsense notions translated into resources for inquiry? Apple is asserting the relevance of her conceptions of the way laymen think about illness over the investigation of the conceptions laymen use. She remains somewhat seduced by the superiority of a medical model of explanation.

This ... does not assume that the lay diagnoses are correct. The only medically valid statement which can be made ... is that the persons depicted are not in the best of health. (Apple, 1960, p. 221)

... whatever the number of correct health facts which the participants knew ... there were some important non-medical characteristics of the kind of health problem which they considered to be illness ... (Apple, 1960, p. 225)

Here again she holds out the myth of a 'correct' diagnosis of which lay versions are merely irrational parodies. Medical practitioners possess truth; laymen, error.

Baumann uses content analysis techniques on responses to a question about what 'most people' mean by being healthy. This is interesting, since most work in this area has tended to concentrate on explaining illness as if it were something separate from health. It parallels attempts to explain crime separately from conformity. Deviance and normality, I shall argue later, must be capable of being accounted for within the same explanatory framework. But for the present let us concentrate on the detail of this study. Firstly, we must note that content analysis does not solve the problem of equivalence. We still have a researcher examining a bundle of data in an attempt to organise them into some kind of theoretical form which still bears an unknown relationship to the actors' theories. The data are treated as a literal description of a state of affairs and the process by which they are produced is ignored. While the three orientations towards health that Baumann has identified may be plausible, and her method for producing them may follow Berelson's (1952) instructions on content analysis to the letter, they have still been produced independently of the methods used by laymen to produce these descriptions of the world. So we are very much in the dark about what these may mean and how we may legitimately make use of them, and there is no way of remedying this situation.

This chapter, then, has outlined some of the principal characteristics of the traditional approaches to the problem of illness and its consequences within medical sociology. I have argued that this research tends to be absolutist and scientistic and that this severely limits its ability to inform us about the nature of human social conduct. Medical sociology has worked within a version of the social world derived from official medical practitioners and has treated this definition itself as unproblematic. The integrity of the lay beliefs that sick people use as guides to their actions has been violated and reduced to pathological irrationality. Once we cease to regard action as essentially rational, in its own context and by its own standards, it inevitably appears perplexing and inexplicable. One particular deficiency has been that medical sociology has failed to develop any conception of illness as a social phenomenon. Clinicians' accounts have been taken over in a relatively uncritical fashion. Since these bear no known relationship to the experience of sick people, they cannot advance our understanding of illness as social conduct. A *biology* of illness is complementary to a *sociology* of illness and in no way a substitute for it. Each has an autonomous realm of practice and an autonomous realm of problems. Once we accept this our attention is directed towards a more pluralist approach to social life.

The search for more adequate intellectual foundations for our enterprises should not, however, blind us to the genuine practical contributions that the orthodox traditions have made to public welfare. My concern to provide a more rigorous theoretical basis for our investigations does not stem from a desire to repudiate social intervention and social concern, but from a desire to improve on what has gone before, in the knowledge that absolutist approaches have had important palliative effects, but have created as many problems as they have solved. I am thinking here particularly of the notion that social equality necessarily entails uniformity of treatment for all citizens. If we recognise the plural nature of our society more clearly we may be able to realise that equality demands a considerable degree of diversity in service provisions. The value of the proposals set out here will ultimately be judged not merely by their theoretical critiques of their predecessors, but by the contribution they can make to the public good.

2 Illness as Social Action

Any break with tradition is necessarily less radical and less decisive than it might appear. We are, after all, to some degree inevitably creatures of the past; we cannot wipe it away but merely seek ways of living with it. So it would obviously be an arrogant claim to suggest that the ideas formulated in this text are entirely new or that they do not rest on the work of a variety of predecessors. However, it is necessary to go beyond those earlier arguments in developing a more adequate account of illness and I now see many of them as less decisive breaks with tradition than they appeared at the time. Rainwater, Strauss and Freidson have all made striking and significant contributions in the past and it would be naive to deny their importance. In particular, their work has pointed us towards a conception of illness as social *action* rather than as mere *behaviour*. This approach has resulted in actors and their conduct being less readily seen as mere puppets moved by the prodding of environmental stimuli or reified attitudes and percepts. These writers present us with a view of conduct as intentional, purposive-rational action. Yet in sociology, as in any other field, too slavish an adherence to the received word will impede rather than advance.

Through my debate with these authors, I want to bring the reader towards a recognition that for sociologists there can be no such things as 'essential illnesses'; rather there are sets of socially organised events organised by members of a collectivity into categories of experience to which the identification 'illness' is accorded. These have no necessary relationship to any biological happening. Biology is seen to fall into a separate domain of explanation governed by a corpus of knowledge in which life scientists have particular rights. If we want to explain how and why people relate to their bodies in certain ways and embark on particular courses of action, we need to examine the relation between biological events and the ways in which they are construed by members of a collectivity in the light of the theories about health and illness available to them. A prime task of the medical sociologist is, then, the study of how both lay persons and 'professionals' theorise about the human body and its operations and management. From the point of view of the sociologist, all such theories have an equal epistemological status. Taken in context they are all equally sensible, rational and reasonable. This does not commit us to regarding them as equally efficacious in achieving actors' goals, although means-ends relationships are themselves social phenomena. The achievement of some goal is itself a social judgement. Nor does it commit us to a view of the total independence of the social and the biological. Our physical condition may impose its own relevance in constraining our possible courses of action. The nature of the possibilities that are opened or closed, however, remains a social product.

The Culture of Poverty

There have been a number of attempts to incorporate cultural factors under the auspices of the more orthodox tradition discussed in the previous chapter. Particular examples can be found in the work of Zborowski (1952) and of Zola, which I reviewed above. In the present context, however, the first serious attempts to use cultural explanations for illness behaviour in the manner for which I am arguing are to be found in the writing of Rainwater (1968) and Strauss (1969). They focussed on the cultural gap between low-status users and professional medical practitioners to explain the low take-up rate of official medical facilities by the poor. Rainwater argued that the very poor - America's Lumpenproletariat - had a distinctive culture. In particular, they held their bodies in low esteem and had relatively low levels of scientific knowledge about medical events. For them, poor health was just one of a number of everyday crises. Their poverty obliged them to seek attention from public health clinics where they were likely to receive curt and cursory treatment. Since this group's conception of ill health was relatively unsophisticated by the standards of scientific medicine and their treatment at clinics deterred them from consultation, medical attention was sought only when social functioning had become severely impaired. Strauss's work, on the other hand, dealt more with the stable working class. He contrasted their life-styles with the life-styles of those towards whom official medical services were geared and noted the difficulties that were likely to be encountered in obtaining satisfactory care from a culturally alien organisation. He concluded that the low levels of consultation among the working class were a function of four main factors:

(i)   a lesser emphasis on health as a worthwhile life-goal;

(ii)   a lesser knowledge about both the nature of illness and the availability of medical care services;

(iii)   the difficulties of access to professional care;

(iv)   their dislike of the official medical system, engendered by the prejudices of professional staff towards them, the stigma of 'charity' attached to publicly provided services and the cultural antipathy to bureaucratic organisation.

Both of these papers are deeply rooted in an exclusively American context (it is not apparent, for example, that there is any sizeable group in the United Kingdom that could be compared with the poor depicted by Rainwater); and both are also rather lacking in systematic empirical evidence. Both Rainwater and Strauss cite others' work to a limited degree, but the central thrust of their accounts has no very clear origin. In Rainwater's case, for example, one might deduce that his account is based on his field work in St Louis, but he does not show anywhere how the account he offers bears on any field data - there are no accounts of his sources of information or extracts from field notes to document his analysis.

But both papers are important in their clear recognition of the plurality of cultures in industrial societies and their avoidance of the absolutist assumption that there is a monolithic version of illness behaviour shared by all but individual deviants with some pathological mental aberration. I shall return to my points of disagreement with their analysis in discussing Freidson's work, but we can note here the basic problems with 'culture of poverty' approaches. Keddie (1973, pp.7-19) has noted how failure to participate in what a minority has succeeded in defining as the 'mainstream' culture of our society has come to be viewed as 'cultural deprivation'. This operates as a euphemism for saying that working class and ethnic groups have a culture inferior to the bourgeois culture that is expressed through our major social institutions. The failure of 'deprived groups' to take full advantage of major institutions such as health services is still seen as located in their background and their inferior knowledge. Any suggestion that their conduct may be a response to organisational arrangements or the behaviour of health workers may still be discounted as irrational. My position is that such conduct is a failure of rationality only from one point of view, one standard of rational conduct that of the investigator. However bizarre their conduct may seem, most people most of the time are able to produce what seem to them 'good' reasons, adequate justifications, which render that conduct rational in its own context.

This cultural perspective may also tend to view social actors as 'cultural dopes' who merely reproduce features of an external and reified culture. It is hard to avoid talking about culture as if it were a concrete object rather than as a term that does not refer to anything with any material existence. Goodenough expresses this view particularly clearly:

> ... culture is not a material phenomenon; it does not consist of things, people, behavior or emotions. It is rather an organisation of these things. It is the forms of things that people have in mind, their models for perceiving, relating and otherwise interpreting them. As such, the things people say and do, their social arrangements and events are products or by-products of their culture as they apply it to the task of perceiving and dealing with their circumstances . . . it is obviously impossible to describe a culture properly simply by describing behavior or social, economic and ceremonial events and arrangements as observed material phenomena. What is required is to construct a theory of the conceptual models which they represent and of which they are artifacts. (Goodenough, 1964, p.36)

'Culture' is sociologists' shorthand for the sets of ideas that social actors appear to be drawing on to generate and interpret actions. As such, it does not have any clear determining part in particular actions, although it obviously shapes the possibilities available. But these possibilities, as we saw in the earlier example of the sheets on the bed in a burning house, are equally influenced by the actor's interests and by his purposes, both of which engage with the body of knowledge and ideas available to him to create the structure of relevant objects, people and events within which action is formed. People are not epiphenomena, mere reflections of their culture; they act to create and re-create that culture.

The Social Construction of Illness

It is Freidson (1971) who offers us for the first time a fully developed attempt to provide a sociology of illness and to articulate this with the study of illness behaviour and, indeed, the sociology of medicine in general. This forms the major theme of the third section of his work on the profession of medicine where he seeks to link the activities of the medical profession and their patients through an account of the social nature of illness.

He argues that the medical profession has obtained virtually exclusive jurisdiction over determining what illness is and how it is to be recognised. By virtue of this authority, medicine creates a legitimate set of possible definitions available within our society to identify someone's actions as 'illness'. Using criteria shaped by its interests, medicine selects and orders biological reality to create a distinct social reality of illness. Freidson regards illness as a form of deviance from some concept of normality: it is both biological deviance and social deviance with distinct biological and social consequences. The biological event and its outcomes may be invariant, but the social event and its consequences are set within a cultural context. Medical knowledge is thought to tap that biological reality and provide stable and objective knowledge. Many sociologists have been misled into taking that for granted and studying the way social factors complicate medically diagnosed illnesses. But, as Freidson points out, medical knowledge is a social construct just as much as any other form of knowledge. It is historically and culturally situated and, judged by external scientific standards of verifiability or reliability, internally heterogeneous. Scientific medicine is irrelevant to the sociologist's concern with meaningful human action. The important topics for him are the meanings given by individuals to illness and the way these meanings influence their behaviour. Illness, then, becomes a form of deviance thought to have a biological origin and to require biological treatment.

Freidson seeks to analyse illness within the paradigm of the sociology of deviance, adopting Becker's (1963) concept of deviance as rule-breaking behaviour. Any study of such behaviour has to take account both of the social rules or norms that are being violated (and their origins), and of the ways in which others perceive and designate acts as rule-breaking. He then takes up Lemert's (1951) distinction between primary and secondary deviation. Primary deviations are individual idiosyncrasies that can be accommodated within the normal performance of a social role, while secondary deviations themselves become roles, part of the social structure. Lemert suggests that secondary deviations develop out of primary ones through a process of interaction between the individual and others, a process that can go on independently of any motivation on the part the individual and any 'objective' initial deviation. Societal reaction is particularly important in our pluralistic society where the applied by regulatory agencies are generated by special groups with particular political access. Illness, according to Freidson, may be either primary or secondary deviance, modifying performance of everyday roles or constituting an organised role in its own right. He goes on to propose a taxonomy of deviance. This is based on ordinary criteria of logical exclusiveness, and places in their historical and cultural contexts the social meanings that are imputed to biological events. The classification is assembled through a critical elaboration of Parsons' concept of the sick role.

Parsons (1951) observes that in modern Western societies 'illness' is used to describe unmotivated deviance that is remediable by the application of rational knowledge owned by a special class of persons. The sufferer is required to adopt successively a 'sick role' and a 'patient role'. In the sick role he is not held responsible for his deviance and is legitimately exempted from normal obligations on condition that he seeks competent help and co-operates with treatment. The deviant is socially isolated and prevented from establishing the desirability of sickness as a moral state. Freidson notes that aspects of the sick role (particularly absolution from responsibility for one's condition) are relevant in analysing a wide range of cultures, not just those found in modern Western societies. He comments, too, that exemption from normal obligations is variable in degree and is itself dependent on the perceived seriousness of the condition. With these two dimensions - imputed responsibility and imputed seriousness - Freidson derives a typology of deviance, which is further modified by the addition of a dimension of legitimacy. He proposes that this categorisation can be used for a processual analysis of illness careers by movement between its six cells, as illustrated by his example of polio victims.

The discussion then turns to the construction of concepts of illness, beginning with a consideration of the concepts of professionals. Freidson notes the institutional division of labour between the various professions in the management of deviance and contemporary changes in this structure, particularly the spread of interpretations of deviance as illness. The medical profession has exclusive jurisdiction over the application of the label of 'illness' and over deciding what is to count as 'illness'. Its commitment to intervention, rather than merely to study or description, leads to a search for sickness. Given the moral nature of this task, doctors become a form of moral entrepreneur (Becker, 1963, pp.147-63). Freidson points out, however, that there is considerable variation in what any diagnosis might be, noting how this is made possible by the priority given to individual clinical experience. Given the importance of placebo effects on both patient and physician, a wide range of possible diagnoses can quite readily be sustained in practice. This may be amplified by the selection processes involved in consultation - selection by the practitioner or self-selection by clients in defining their condition. We may find both under-reporting (by clients) and over-reporting (by professionals imputing greater significance to a condition than its true incidence warrants). Freidson is suspicious of the value of true incidence studies, in any case, since they are based on categories generated by medical practice rather than by social functioning.

We then turn to a discussion of the lay construction of illness. Freidson observes that the implementation of professional constructions depends upon the perception by laymen that they have an illness serious enough to require professional help and for which such help is likely to have a relevant treatment. In a simple society this is not a problem, since folk practitioners merely specialise in what everybody knows. But in modern societies, where there is a responsible profession, there is a monopoly of an esoteric body of knowledge of which the layman is largely ignorant. There is thus an inevitable gap between the conceptions of laymen and professionals. Entry to professional care is the outcome of a social process whose critical variables are lay conceptions of sickness and the structure of lay social life. Freidson discusses the influence of cultural perceptions of pain as an example of initial distress and the significance of social meanings rather than biological events. He goes on to examine the ways in which deviations from a normal state of health are recognised in the context of everyday experience through the distinction between primary and secondary deviation. Laymen and physicians ascribe differing importances to different events. A conception of illness implies participation in a cultural system of health knowledge. Freidson describes the inadequacies of this knowledge in lower-class people. They are ignorant about bodily functions, hold medically unfashionable theories about remedies and have a concrete notion of normality based on how they feel rather than the more abstract self-evaluation of the better educated. The discussion then turns to the organisation of the entrance to care. Freidson regards the social structure as central to this. In particular, it includes a lay referral system which is culturally and structurally defined, and through which individuals are processed into some form of care. Various types of network are described and related to their cultural contexts. A lay referral career is also shaped by the dimensions of seriousness, responsibility and legitimacy described above.

Through this lay system, individuals are brought into professional management, in which the physician will seek to reorganise his client's experience in medical terms, to determine what is 'really' wrong and persuade him to accept the proper 'scientific' treatment. Freidson describes some of the elements that are likely to be involved in this process in the context of both institutional and ambulatory care. He identifies various possible patterns of relationship between doctor and patient along a dimension of the relative activity or passivity of each party. These various structures of medical activity represent the career of being a sick person.

Some Critical Observations

I have summarised at some length Freidson's account of the social construction of illness. This reflects in large measure his own exhaustive discussion of the literature in this area. It accords too with the influence this formulation has had on recent thinking in medical sociology, although it has perhaps been slightly overshadowed by his discussion of functional autonomy and its consequences for the social organisation of medical practice. But a summary of this length is necessary also to bring out the points of detail at which, I shall argue, Freidson's account becomes inadequate and which, taken together, require important modifications of his model. In part, these disagreements arise from the contrast between Freidson's emphasis on a moral critique of the activities of the medical profession and my own emphasis on the need for a sounder theoretical framework for the understanding of social action. In that sense it may be argued that it is slightly unfair to subject Freidson's work to detailed textual scrutiny, and in the context of the author's apparent intentions there is some justice in this criticism. However, I would suggest that the work has had an impact on medical sociology going beyond the force of moral criticism and that it is thus entirely appropriate to treat the work as a theoretical enterprise and to ask questions about the nature of that enterprise.

My basic contention is that Freidson has been insufficiently willing to make a radical break with traditional work in this field and that this approach, rather than being definitive, should be regarded as transitional between the orthodox functionalism that has provided what theoretical backbone most medical sociology has had and the ethnoscientific approach that I shall be presenting. Accordingly, I shall begin by specifying the problems I find in Freidson's account. These centre around his view of the concepts of knowledge and of social structure, with consequential effects on other elements such as the concepts of lay referral network and the sick role.

The perspective adopted by Freidson bears an important and self-avowed debt to the work of interactionist theorists of deviance, notably Becker and Lemert, but one of the difficulties of discussing this group is the heterogeneity of their thought, as Goode (1975) shows. In the context of social deviance, interactionism, labelling theory or whatever we may like to call it, is less a theory than a perspective, a way of looking at things rather than a way of explaining them. The unity of this approach is as much an artefact of its critics as of a clear intellectual convergence. Nevertheless, this approach has come to display a number of features that can be profitably examined and built on, although these are not necessarily shared by a delimited body of workers under the auspices of a clear paradigm. In criticising interactionist/labelling theories of deviance I am concentrating on Freidson's particular synthesis and the version of other theorists portrayed through his work, rather than the perspective as a whole. That would be well beyond the proper scope of this book.

One of the main contributions of these approaches to deviance has been their break with notions of objective deviance; the notion that certain phenomena are inevitably and necessarily deviant. As Warren and Johnson (1972) contend, however, this is not the same as saying that they had adopted a fully pluralist view of social phenomena. Although they had discarded the functionalist monolith of a unitary and homogeneous social structure whose participants acted under the aegis of exterior, reified values, they had replaced it by a model that merely substituted plural value systems while retaining their deterministic relation to social action. Zimmerman and Wieder (1971) set out a similar argument in their general critique of the interactionist position. While the interactionists viewed social structures as a symbolic rather than an existentially real order, the effect was merely to push reification back one stage further. The study of the use of values to produce an observable and experientially real social order, through their invocation by actors to render intelligible the acts of others and to produce intelligible acts themselves, was neglected. As Douglas (1970, p.12) concluded, the interactionists had made the breakthrough of envisaging as problematic the processes of categorisation by which members of a society imputed morality or immorality, health or illness to one another. However, the process was merely affirmed and, as Blum (1970, p.39n) notes, used as the basis of a moral critique rather than being examined as a topic.

Warren and Johnson go on to argue that labelling theorists tended to concentrate on acts rather than actors, studying the ways acts were assembled into careers of primary and secondary deviation as actors took up deviant roles. They use Becker's (1963) account of becoming a marihuana user, for example, to show that he identifies the identity transformation of the user with a sequence of acts. Actually, I think they are a little confused here. What Becker is doing here is to present a somewhat abstracted and idealised description of the careers of marihuana users. The point that is really at issue is the degree to which this does or does not work as a second-order typification, that is a typification of the typifications actually used by individuals. Since Becker does not really present the kind of data on individuals' careers and their courses of action in practical situations which would allow us to warrant his abstraction as being clearly connected in some way with observable events, his account inevitably comes through as a series of decontextualised acts. In terms of Becker's interests this is fair enough, and to suggest that it is merely a question of acts and actors skirts the real issue about the relationship between theory and data. This is a general problem with interactionism and cannot be discussed in depth here. However, broadly, it can be argued that interactionism has a tendency to substitute glosses of events for analyses of them. In other words its practitioners redescribe events in their own fashion rather than analysing participants' descriptions of them; field data, for example, tend to offer us descriptions of interaction rather than the interaction itself.

The labelling theorists also tended to emphasise the role of official agencies in the labelling process, tending to regard lay cultures, where they were involved, as defective, a point I discuss at more length later. Thus, they tended to continue to operate with official, absolutist categorisations of deviance and deviant acts rather than to analyse everyday notions of deviation. Their selection of areas for discussion, for example, involved according the same unquestioned status to official categories as I am arguing medical sociologists have accorded to Western professional medical categories. Labelling involved public acts by rule-enforcers rather than the whole set of contingencies of everyday life. This over-reliance on official definitions led, even within a pluralistic model, towards notions of 'real' deviance that could be legislated by the sociologist independently of the social meanings applied by the other participants in the events he was studying to the events in question. None of this, of course, is to suggest that official agencies and public acts of rule-enforcement are not themselves everyday activities, as Warren and Johnson seem to imply at times. But their study presents a partial and misleading picture if it is separated from the study of everyday life. The sociological understanding of 'deviance' depends upon the sociological understanding of the practical accomplishments of morality and immorality in everyday affairs.

Freidson continues to operate squarely within this interactionist tradition. His notion of social order contains persistent ambiguities between objective and subjective notions. At times he seems to be positing some kind of out-there social reality and to be working within a normative paradigm depicting social action as directed by exterior values; at others, he views social reality as an intersubjective construction produced out of the interpretive work and social theories of society members. We can see this in the contrast between the two following passages. In the first Freidson is talking about a profession as something that can be unequivocally legislated by the sociologist. It is a tangible phenomenon to which the accounts of society members are irrelevant. In the second, he seems to be hinting more at a view of 'profession' as a category applied as an outcome of interpretive work.

... whether or not an occupation is a profession is established by the analysis of the relation of occupations to one another in the social structure ... by defining a profession structurally ... one can, without embarrassment or apology, deal with the difference between what a group typically claims its members to be as opposed to what they are, and between what is generally believed about a group and what is actually the case. (Freidson, 1971, p.186)

They have also come to create their own conception of themselves as professions and to see their conceptions adopted by outsiders, including sociologists, to represent what professionals actually are rather than what professionals think they are or claim to be. (Freidson, 1971, p.380)

I have discussed Freidson's concept of profession more fully elsewhere (Dingwall, 1974, 1976, 1977), but we can find similar ambiguities in the context of the present study. For example, in the following passage, having defined social structure as 'an organisation of people's relations each to the other', he goes on to talk about how this organisation can enforce particular ideas about sickness:

Indeed social structure can force people to act sick even though they may not believe themselves to be sick. Usually, however, the individual has internalised the views of his associates and he is likely to behave 'spontaneously' the way he is supposed to. (Freidson, 1971, p.289)

In the space of a few lines he slides from a sentence that can be understood as implying a social order constructed out of social interaction, to one based upon the internalisation of an external system and an external culture. This position is, of course, quite understandable in the light of Freidson's polemical concerns, but I would argue that it is unsatisfactory for a sociological analysis.

Freidson's out-there social structure is not, however, a homogeneous one after the functionalist model. He recognises the relevance of cultural pluralism in restricting the applicability of much of his analysis to the American white Protestant middle class (Freidson, 1971, pp.224-43). However, his plural groups remain puppets of their values.

The use of this type of concept of social structure has two important consequences, relating to the status of concepts like 'sick role' and 'lay referral network' and to the view that Freidson adopts of the knowledge of medical and non-medical personnel. His principal criticisms of the Parsonian notion of the sick role are empirical, that it does not exhaust the available universe of possibilities of illness activities and that it is hortatory rather than analytical. He proposes a more elaborated model set into a processual account of illness careers. Yet this model retains the same logical form. The roles are scripted by the sociologist and played by the actors. One can however argue, with Cicourel (1973, pp.11-40), that roles are merely sense-assembly devices. The concept of the sick role, in whatever version, relies upon a notion of an internalised normative system which provides prescriptive rules for role-playing. But as Cicourel notes, this account cannot deal with the phenomenon of innovation. Just as speakers can produce grammatically correct novel utterances, so can persons produce socially correct novel conduct. He proposes an alternative approach founded on the articulation of action settings with cognitive senses of social structure, which enable the actor to assign meaning to the setting and to identify and order the relevance of its constituent object-events. This sense of social structure is developmental. It constitutes the setting, in the light of the actor's socially distributed knowledge about the nature of phenomena, and is constituted by the setting, and the limitations that co-participants or material objects place on it. Thus we can seek to determine how general rules or norms are drawn upon to produce or evaluate a course of action and how their contextual use provides for evolutionary change. The identification of a line of conduct as a role is conditional upon the methods employed by the actor to generate behaviour that he regards as sensible and those employed by the observer to evaluate the sense of the actor's conduct. Thus the description of a role is unavoidably opaque in its relation to everyday social life, unless it provides for the formulation and recognition of 'appropriate' conduct by actor and observer. The concepts of role-playing outlined by Parsons and Freidson provide for the formulation of the sick role as a sociologist's concept. But it remains impossible to say what relation, if any, such a concept bears to the concepts used by members of a collectivity to render each other's conduct intelligible. And it is these everyday activities that are important for the understanding of meaningful social interaction.

Similar objections may be levelled against the notion of a lay 'referral network'. This is likewise a sociologists' *post hoc* construct, imposing a form and structure on a series of events that bears no contingent relationship to the procedures whereby this series of events was produced. Freidson again displays the somewhat ambiguous relationship between the subjective and the objective that we have already noted. Lay referral networks have both cultural and structural dimensions. But in both instances these are out-there phenomena which are external to the activities of individual actors, existing in some inexplicable, self-evident form. According to this model, structural features can somehow directly enforce particular views of illness, although enforcement is usually unnecessary since an internalised culture produces the appropriate behaviour 'spontaneously'. Sufferers are processed through the network to a variety of outcomes. This view does have the merit of accounting for a variety of courses of action - professional help, folk help, self-medication, etc. - but it is again divorced from any firm foundation in the interpretive work of the sick person and the choices that serially confront him. In Manning's words, 'It is my alternative contention that the network itself is *created* by the search, *located* by the searching, *defined* via the transactions carried on between the knowledgeable informants (referees), the abortionists and self-defined candidates and begins to function as a result of the actor's involvement in it.' (Manning, 1971, p. 144). Social networks are not just *there,* they are devices employed by sociologists to order actors' conduct. Barnes, the originator of the term, has always been clear about this:

> Where possible I shall suggest ways of measuring characteristics, not only because this is one way of giving precision and comparability to our enquiries, but also because it is easier to argue about quantified concepts. *They can be clearly seen for what they really are, analytical constructs and not mistaken for Platonic essences.* (Barnes, 1969, p.54, my emphasis)

Freidson's problems are in part related to the second principal difficulty I identified in his analysis - the different status he accords to scientific medical and folk medical knowledge. As Warren and Johnson noted, although the deviance theorists saw official conceptions of deviance as part of their problem, they continued to work within them. Similarly, although Freidson views medical knowledge as part of his problem he does not see it as problematic. Thus, he continues to operate within medical categories of disease thought to derive from a body of knowledge that has some privileged status - scientific medicine. Although he recognises the problems involved in labelling medical knowledge as scientific at present, in view of its incoherence and heterogeneous logic, it has that possibility and is, thereby, in some sense 'better' than folk or lay knowledge.

It is not at all clear that this is a tenable position. I shall be arguing that there is no sharp distinction between scientific and commonsense knowledge, but that they are continuous and separated only by the different warrants required to justify everyday and scientific theorising. As Scott (1968, p.180) has said, 'rational descriptions reside in the human communities in which they are made'. Medical knowledge is judged in terms of the standards of the medical community and warranted as rational in the light of their standards of rationality. Since most doctors do not have to think in theoretical terms in most of their everyday practice, their knowledge inevitably has a somewhat commonsensical character. However, even if official medical knowledge were scientific - in the sense that it was invoked solely by scientific theorisers - this would still give us no sociological grounds for according it a superior status. One might wish to argue that it was more efficacious, but standards of efficacy are themselves situated within theoretical systems that provide for the recognition of what is to count as a problem, what are relevant ways of tackling it and what is to count as a solution. Thus I would argue that it is fundamentally a mistake to treat the health knowledge of laymen or folk practitioners as a defective version of official medical knowledge, as Freidson does when, for example, he describes laymen as 'comparatively ignorant ... [with] antiquated notions ... unfashionable ideas' (Freidson, 1971, pp.287-8).

A good example of the limitations of this kind of thinking is Lewis's (1975) account of illness among the Gnau. His account is directed towards assessing the distance by which their thinking falls short of that of Westernised medicine. As a qualified physician, as well as an anthropologist, Lewis sees himself in a position to specify the objective nature of their illnesses:

> The independent medical assessment of their sicknesses makes it possible to indicate what burden or severity of misfortune they respond to. The medical nature of an illness and the social response to it are interrelated. Without knowing the medical condition, it must remain partly uncertain which aspects

of response have social or cultural roots rather than follow directly from the changes induced by disease. My present aim then is to make clear what medical conditions I observed so that they may later be matched against the responses to them. The account in this chapter takes the observer's viewpoint and attempts to define objectively the amount and severity of their illnesses. (Lewis, 1975, pp. 95-6)

While the Gnau's medical knowledge is socially situated and represents the application of their own classificatory system to the world that is available for perception, Lewis's is a direct copy of that perceptual world. Yet it is not at all clear upon what grounds such a claim can be upheld. How can Lewis demonstrate that his knowledge is truer than that of the Gnau, other than in the context of a set of cultural assumptions that the Gnau do not share? Western medical knowledge and Gnau medical knowledge are equally true, for Westerners and the Gnau respectively. Lewis's claim to objectivity is merely an assertion of Western absolutism. His failure to break with this stance is behind much of the disappointment that his account engenders. Despite its meticulous observation of the Gnau, its assumption throughout of the superiority of Western thought leaves it standing very palely beside the sophistication of some of the work discussed in the final chapter. It is particularly noteworthy, for example, how he misses the significance of Frake's work on illness among the Subanun. I shall return to this point later.

My general concern in this chapter, then, has been to define more clearly the differences between the position that I am taking up in this work and a number of similar positions that have been adopted in the past. I discussed some of the difficulties presented by various theories of cultural deprivation, culture deficit or cultural poverty. The questions here must always be: deprived of *what* culture, deficient by *whose* standards, impoverished by *what* comparison? Some of these issues were revived in considering the seminal work of Eliot Freidson. Medical sociology has been severely handicapped by the lack of attention it has received from the major theorists - Marx, Weber, Durkheim and G. H. Mead all passed over this theme. Parsons was the first major writer to give serious attention to the field, and Freidson's work is arguably the first of comparable significance since. As with Parsons', so too has Freidson's account set the terms of debate for a generation of medical sociologists. And it is precisely because of this impact that it demands detailed scrutiny.

I have however sought to show that there are certain serious ambiguities in some key portions of Freidson's analysis. In particular, he seems uncertain about the factual status that he wishes to accord to social phenomena. This gives rise to a tendency to abstract concepts like culture and social structure from the occasions when they are used and somehow to set them up as external to social actors. Consequently, Freidson's actors become reduced to cultural dopes: they no longer create and use their culture but are created and used by it. Secondly, Freidson tends to treat Western scientific knowledge as more valid than other kinds of knowledge. Furthermore, while expert theories are seen as part of the problem, they are not made problematic in the same way as lay knowledge. In this he resembles other interactionist theorists of deviance who made rule-breaking a problem without considering the prior topic - the practical use of those rules in the first place. I suspect that both of these difficulties arise out of Freidson's primary concern with moral criticism and his need to secure a foundation for his evaluation of American medicine. My purposes here are different and, to satisfy them, some alternative approach is required.

We have seen how a plural vision of social order does not necessarily lead its authors into a pluralist version of sociology. The remainder of this book will argue that our future inquiries should be pointed in that direction and will attempt to suggest what it might look like.

3   Accounts of Illness

Thus far, we have concentrated on the ways in which medical sociologists have looked at the traditional topic of illness behaviour and the various formulations and reformulations they have proposed. I have suggested that these inquiries have had a predominantly pragmatic motive and have concentrated upon the question, 'Who uses official medical services?' rather than the question, 'How do people come to feel ill and what do they do about it?'. Some reasons have been suggested for the bias towards regarding illness as a social rather than a sociological problem, relating both to the practical constraints on medical sociologists and to their own humane concerns. In the next chapter I shall move on towards the development of an alternative model cast in more strictly sociological terms. Before doing this, however, I want to pursue further the issues of the relative status of scientific and folk medical knowledge and their respective models of rationality. In doing this I shall also take the opportunity to examine more deeply some of the answers that have been proposed to the question, 'What is illness?'.

Fabrega (1972, 1974) notes how many of the difficulties that arise in talking about disease arise from the sheer variety of ways in which the word can be used at both syntactic and semantic levels. He proposes that the term 'disease' can be used in the following ways:

1.   As an abstract general term, purporting to refer to each or any of the members of the class of 'disease'. That includes hypertension, diabetes, etc. For example (a) 'Diseases found in this community tend to be more serious'. (b) 'Diseases due to bacteria have always plagued mankind'. In each instance the term *diseases* functions as a general abstract term. However, the meaning provided by the context of each sentence differs, serving to narrow the focus of the term: (a) a subgroup of diseases that are serious and (b) any and all diseases caused by bacteria.

2.   With a singularising modifier [e.g. a, the] purporting to refer to exactly one thing. For example, 'That disease has an abrupt onset' or 'the disease that he has'. In these instances, the term with the

41

singularising modifier together function as an abstract singular term.

Two different and independent manners of classifying the term follow:

3.   As a denotative term, purporting to *refer* to things. For example:
      'The disease had an abrupt onset'. Here the abstract general term
      disease is conjoined with a singularising modifier *the* and forms a
      denotative term that refers to a specific disease [i.e. it can be
      substituted as an abstract version of any particular disease name].
4.   As an attributive term, purporting to *apply* to things. For example:
      'You could see that he was diseased'. In this instance, the term is
      used to qualify things [i.e. to describe qualities of the phenomena
      under discussion]. (Fabrega, 1974, p.123)

At times, then, the term can suggest either the existence of an abstract entity
grounded in the concrete world or a quality or property that people take on or
acquire or a concrete entity located in time and space.

It is important to remember that there is no object or concrete thing that
is a disease, although we may sometimes talk as if there is. As Wittgenstein
(1972) suggests, this involves breaking with the idea that using a sentence
involves imagining something for every word. He notes that we calculate with
words, translating them now into one picture, now into another; words are not
necessarily accompanied by unique images. What we have in the present case
is a collection of biological events to which the term 'disease' may be applied
under certain conditions. The application of this term is a move in a language
game, part of a form of life. A form of life is the commonsense social
knowledge of the player, which in this case allows him to recognise these
events as constituting a disease and at the same time enables him to warrant
or justify this identification by reference to them. Like any other socially
organised account, disease terms have a reflexive character: the production
of recognisably adequate accounts of events depends upon the producer's and
the hearers' knowledge of the settings in which those events are located.
These settings are, in turn, constituted out of those same recognisably
adequate accounts (Garfinkel, 1967, pp.7-10). This should, I suggest, lead us
towards conceiving of 'disease' and 'illness' as ascriptions to events that take
place under certain specifiable conditions, rather than seeing them as marks
that bind objects and events unequivocally together.

It is also important to remember that 'disease' can in principle be
distinguished from 'natural variation', although in practice the drawing of

distinctions between the two may be a debatable matter. Nevertheless, both terms are recognisable and recognisably counterposed. 'Disease' as a term, then, both evaluates and implies a need for correction when it is ascribed to any set of events. These events are held up as undesirable and as requiring remedy. (At this point some of the convergences with and distinctions from the sociological term 'deviance' begin to be clarified. I shall return to this point in the following chapter.)

The term 'disease' can, for present purposes, be located within either of two quite distinct theoretical systems. In another terminology we could suggest that it was embedded in two forms of life - we can view it as either a biological or a behavioural disturbance. The two are somewhat separate, although not totally autonomous at this point. It is precisely this lack of autonomy that underlies many of our difficulties, and one of our key tasks is to unravel the two systems at work. In this, I owe much to Fabrega's (1972) discussion.

Disease as a Biological Discontinuity

'Disease' here carries an orthodox medical meaning, namely some abnormality in function and/or structure of any part, process or system of the body. The range of application of the term, or the class of events to which it applies - its extension - would include such events as 'appendicitis', 'hypertension', 'diabetes', 'measles' or 'syphilis'. In any particular instance the term 'disease' can be substituted for or include each or any member of these separate terms.

In a biologically oriented framework the characteristics that define specific diseases refer to biological processes. Information is gathered by means of indicators like X-rays, blood sugar levels, electroencephalograph readings or biopsies, which are thought to tap these biological processes directly. This framework is, then, closely associated with developments in Western science. Lewis (1953) remarks on the way physicians can readily reach a consensus on the operation of body systems by reference to well-defined criteria which are generally familiar to members of the medical profession and which become progressively sharper with advances in scientific knowledge. Differences of opinion are matters that will eventually be superseded by advances in knowledge. A feature of this advance, which Fabrega (1972, p.185) particularly notes, is the gradual elimination of verbal reports as either necessary or sufficient for diagnosis and the aim of biological scientists of dispensing with them altogether: instead of having to rely on subjective verbal reports of symptoms, the medical practitioner will be able to use signs derived from objective indices of biological structure or function regardless of whether the supposed patient actually feels ill.

Viewed in this light, specific diseases can be said to be universal. If the current norms used by physicians to judge biological functioning are reliable and valid, then any indication of a deviation is *prima facie* evidence of disease. This is not quite as straightforward as it sounds however. The development of norms of physical functioning is very difficult. As Lewis (1953, p.113) notes, the range of variability in the human species is very wide and very individual, and no instrument of deceptive precision can remove the difficulty. The physician really has to work out a norm for each patient and develop a rough appraisal of any departure from it. King recounts the story of a precise young physician who had just joined his laboratory and asked King what they considered the normal haemoglobin level of the blood to be.

When I answered, 'Twelve to sixteen grams, more or less', he was very puzzled. Most laboratories, he pointed out, called 15 grams normal, or perhaps 14.5. He wanted to know how, if my norm was so broad and vague, he could possibly tell whether a patient suffered from anemia, or how much anemia. I agreed that he had quite a problem on his hands and that it is a very difficult thing to tell. So difficult, in fact, that trying to be too precise is actually misleading, inaccurate, stultifying to thought, and philosophically very unsound.

He wanted to know why I didn't take one hundred or so normal individuals, determine their hemoglobin by our method, and use the resulting figure as the normal value for our method. This, I agreed, was a splendid idea. But how were we to pick out the normals? The obvious answer is, just take one or two hundred healthy people, free of disease ... But that is exactly the difficulty. We think of health as freedom from disease, and disease as an aberration from health. This is travelling in circles, getting us nowhere. (King, 1954, pp.194-5)

Obviously the biologistic approach to the study of disease has made possible major contributions to the lives of men and women in our society. But these benefits can be exaggerated. Public health has probably been improved more by social change and an increasing standard of living among the working classes. Sanitation, pure water, pure food, anti-pollution legislation and redistribution of wealth are the real conquerors of infectious disease. And, of course, there are the iatrogenic effects of medicine, which

Illich (1975) so graphically describes in considering both the individual damage of medically induced illness and the social damage of the attrition of capacities for facing pain, suffering and death. The price of a materially comfortable life may be the erosion of individual liberty by the social control of medicine and the added suffering of a spiritually barren death. Nevertheless, even Illich does not seek to deny that medical science has been of benefit to individuals, and inclines towards a strengthening of community control over medical practice rather than the annihilation of modern medicine.

We can however locate some fundamental difficulties with this paradigm. Several of these are rather beyond the scope of the present discussion but merit some mention at this point. Firstly, there is the problem of the place of disease in the relationship between man and his biological environment. Scientific medicine has, for the most part, developed against a background of a most unnatural ecological setting for human animals. It seems to be accepted that *homo sapiens* evolved originally in savannah regions as a hunter-gatherer among the scrub, grassland and scattered trees. This is a somewhat different environment from the modern world's cities where medical researchers for the most part live and work. If we follow Dubos's (1965) argument that disease is a phase in the homeostatic relationship between man and his biological environment, then we can see that a disturbed environment is likely to have consequences for the process of homeostasis. In short, are our identifications of human biological disturbance - 'disease' - being judged against a standard of spurious normality based on the adaptation between men and a deviant environment? We could try to remedy this by going to do field work in hunter gatherer societies. But here we have the problem of determining a baseline for our clinical judgements. What is normal variation among these populations and what is to be counted as disease? We cannot simply export our own standards, or we defeat the whole object of the exercise. There are also practical problems. It may be difficult to establish diagnoses without the direct availability of the apparatus of scientific medicine. Indeed, it may be difficult to establish any diagnosis. It is not at all clear to what extent doctors do routinely establish discriminatory diagnoses. The demands of research in a foreign land on a strange population to unfamiliar standards of precision may have some curious effects on the results.

The unavailability of technical aids may lead to a greater reliance on verbal reports, which are still, of course, necessary even within the culture from which the doctor comes. We return to our old friend the problem of equivalence. Consider a physician asking another member of his society about subjective feelings. Does the question, 'Do you feel overtired?' mean the same to an accountant, a fisherman and a miner? How the problems are magnified when the physician is interrogating a member of a totally different way of life.

Finally, we return to the central theme of this book - the relationship between biological events and human action. There is no reason why the 'diseases' of the medical scientist and the 'diseases' of any lay member of his own society, let alone the members of a different society, should be in an isomorphic, one-to-one relation. If we are interested in the social consequences of illness, it is to the social nature of illness to which we must direct our attention.

Disease as a Behavioural Discontinuity

The difficulties of the straightforward application of the biologistic model to the social aspects of illness have been widely recognised in psychiatric illness, where, in part, this reflects the general problem of trying to ascribe 'illness' to a set of conditions that have no clear and direct biological manifestations. (That small number of conditions treated by psychiatrists that do have organic manifestations are probably best regarded as physical illnesses.) The issues raised by applying such a model to psychiatric illness have been exhaustively debated among clinicians and social scientists, and I do not intend to pursue this argument further here, except to note one crucial point. This debate has almost invariably presupposed a split between mind and body, between psychiatric illness and physical illness. As Sedgwick concludes, after noting the considerable accomplishment of scientific psychiatry's critics in demonstrating the limitations of its positivist thinking, '[They] have accomplished the feat of criticising the concept of mental illness without ever examining the (surely more inclusive, and logically prior) concept of illness.' (Sedgwick, 1972, p.12). Even the most recent work, like Coulter's (1974) incisive analysis, begs this question. These biases are not however confined only to studies within our own society, but, as both Sedgwick and Fabrega (1974, pp.39-44) note, extend also to work on non-Western societies. The study of folk medicine, with a few exceptions, *is* the study of folk psychiatry. This bias rests on a set of unexamined assumptions about the universal relevance of Western classifications of organic disease. The cultural context of psychiatric disturbances has been more readily conceded, partly as a result of the debates referred to above and partly as a result of the longstanding interest of anthropologists in the relationship between culture and individual personality. Folk classifications of organic disease have either been ignored or have been reduced to psychiatric illness, psychosomatic epiphenomena of some aberration from the prevailing theories of sanity.

There are two kinds of approach available to the study of the social nature of illness. We can see it either as a behavioural discontinuity or as a phenomenologic discontinuity. In the former approach, disease is treated as a set of changes in behaviour with indicators referring to specific patterns of behaviour. As Fabrega (1972, pp.186-7) shows, the logic of this model closely parallels the logic of a biologistic model. Changes in observable biological function/behaviour are indicated by specific changes in biological/behavioural activities. Where we are dealing with psychiatric illnesses this kind of conception is not uncommon, producing as it does a self-contained theoretical system which does not articulate with any alteration in bodily function. However, the parallelism between the two frames does suggest the possibility of erecting some kind of translation, although it is emphasised that the two frames are not isomorphic. Biological 'diseases' and behavioural 'diseases' *may* be empirically identical but they will not have the same indicators, since these lie in separate realms of phenomena; nor will they refer to the same universe of deviation and normality.

Engel (1960) has developed one possible translation model that seeks to integrate behavioural and biological diseases. He attacks the assumption that disease is a thing in itself, unrelated to the sufferer and his situation and caused by some external, malevolent influence, a single defective part or an occult internal force. The difficulties of this search for monocausal explanations have however been compounded by the influence of nosology, the demand for the naming and classification of diseases. Naming often takes place along irrelevant dimensions of the condition, which may impede creative ways of researching the disease and give a spurious impression of certainty. Names for diseases are often derived from those features that are most immediately obvious, or were at some point in the past, rather than from those that are the most important clinically. Engel cites the examples of pernicious anaemia, which is not simply a disease of the blood and is no longer pernicious, and *lupus erythematosus disseminatus,* which is not a skin disease and is not disseminated. While the understanding of conditions is always changing, names seldom do, and their connotations for the physician may constitute stumbling blocks for advances in explanation or therapy. Diagnostic labels are shorthand descriptions of a bundle of information, rather than complete and exhaustive definitions of illness. In arriving at a diagnosis a physician employs a great deal of tacit knowledge, which is necessary to the completion of this task but is not manifested in diagnostic activity.

Engel also accepts that disease is a natural phenomenon. Diseases form a part of the routine transactions between man and environment and represent disruptions in the normal balance. The presence of a complaint is presumptive evidence of a disease. This complaint may take the form of a symptom, privately experienced and not necessarily communicated to anyone else, or a sign, outwardly manifested and the subject of attention from others. Since complaints have both internal and external dimensions, the absence of signs or reported symptoms cannot be taken as evidence that a person is not ill. Symptoms may be unrecognised, denied or unreported, or there may be a latent phase in the disease (as in syphilis or shingles). In this model, both symptoms and signs may be either biological or behavioural.

The description of disease as a *scientific* undertaking that Engel proposes is clearly much broader than the traditional description of diseases as the object of a set of activities bounded by the function and role of officially sanctioned physicians. A clear distinction is made between the study of disease as a scientific enterprise and the practice of medicine. Under this umbrella many kinds of processes, like grief, may be thought of as disease since their structure is basically similar. The identification of some of these conditions as 'diseases' and the exclusion of others merely reflects social and scientific conventions.

Engel further argues for the expansion of the study of aetiology beyond the simple question of *how* a disease affects the systems of the body to the further question *why?*, in both its aspects of *how come?* and *what for?* - how did this person come to fall ill with this condition and what are the functions of the changes in body systems consequent upon pathogenic invasion? The origins of disease may lie in the genetic inheritance of individuals or populations, disturbances in organic or psychological development, the presence or absence of physical and chemical elements in the environment, bacteriological agents operating in both individuals and their surroundings and intrinsic or extrinsic psychological stresses. These factors may operate singly or in concert.

Despite the sympathetic echo that there is between many of Engel's arguments and those propounded here from very different intellectual origins, there remain certain difficulties with this conception of disease. I am thinking particularly of the way in which the translation from the biological to the behavioural is accomplished by the adoption of an organismic model of social life, in which social and biological systems are presented as logically continuous. This approach has a long history in social science. Herbert Spencer developed a very elaborate organismic theory based on Darwinian principles, and there are strong elements of organismic thought in Durkheim's work. Nearer our own times, Parsons' work was much influenced by the distinguished biologist L.J. Henderson. This model enjoys a continuing vogue; it is perhaps less fashionable now in mainstream sociology than it has been for some years, although one might regard some of the cybernetically influenced systems theories as the model's latter-day transformations. Outside academic sociology the presence of this way of thinking in the systemic theories of practitioners in a variety of applied disciplines ensures its continued currency as a way of describing social life.

This is not the place for a detailed critique of organismic thought, but I do want to note some of its principal defects. First, there is commonly some confusion about whether the model is to be treated literally or metaphorically. As a metaphor, the position need only be evaluated in heuristic terms as a device for explaining sociological thinking to an outside audience. The major problem, though, is a tendency to take the metaphor literally, to slide from thinking of a society as like an organism to thinking of that society as an organism. The other problems with this model follow from this shift.

Thus, taken literally, the second problem with the organismic model is the fallacy of attributing concreteness to something that does not possess it. Social systems simply do not exist in the same way as biological systems. One may be able to draw some useful analogies between ecological systems and social systems, as the Chicago School did, but a social system is of a completely different ontological order from a living organism. There is a substantial difference between the predicates of 'That is a rat' and 'That is Britain' or 'That is a hospital'. A rat may be thought of as a collection of biological actions; Britain and hospitals are collections of social action. These latter terms do not denote anything with any material existence in the way that a rat exists.

Thirdly, social action is reduced to an epiphenomenon of systemic processes, that is to say social action is depicted as a marginal consequence of processes within the system as a whole. In effect, it becomes assimilated to behaviour generated by a chain of mechanical stimuli and responses. One reaction to incoming signals triggers another and so on until some action emerges from the organism. The processes whereby actors selectively attend to, perceive and interpret incoming signals are depicted as a Newton's Cradle where the impact of the swinging ball at one end detaches another ball at the other. This plainly seems a poor description on the basis of the data available to us on the phenomena of attention and perception. Without reference to the selective and interpretive aspects of the cognitive processes that precede action, collections of social action such as organisations can be only partially understood.

Finally, social action is seen as determined by the need of all systems to drive towards homeostasis. Systems are presented as having inbuilt tendencies towards equilibrium: if the system is disturbed, then there is a drive towards containing that disturbance and restoring balance. This element is particularly strong in Engel's account with its clear Freudian influences. Built-in biological drives press for discharge. If this is not possible, or is realised only in a partial or ineffective fashion, then intrapsychic or social conflict is likely to ensue. Drive theories, instinct theories and similar accounts that rely on unconscious and non-rational motivations are somewhat impervious to systematic inquiry. The combined effects of these functional imperatives and the epiphenomenal nature of action is a highly determinist view of human conduct, playing down any question of will, intention or volition or of structured conflict between plural and competing versions of social order. Although homeostatic models can accommodate individualised variation as a source of wobbles around their equilibrium point, they presuppose a generally unitary and homogeneous view of the society they represent.

In this view of disease as a behavioural discontinuity, then, 'diseases', parallelling the biological model, remain as secondary phenomena of systemic processes. They are still, in some sense, 'out there', although the world 'out-there' is more complex and more sophisticated than the world of the crude monocausalists who are searching for an explanation in terms of some single malevolent intervention. But, in general, we are still confronted by an absolutist codification of disease that avoids the moral issues this phenomenon presents. Behavioural diseases, as much as biological diseases, are specified primarily in terms of sets of behaviour, classified together by the observer without any necessary regard for the classifications of the alleged sufferer. A small class of experts continues to monopolise the right to impose a particular set of socially sanctioned theories on other members of their society. We might concede this right if we were to concede the claim that this body of theory did, indeed, have some privileged status. It is to that claim that our attention now turns.

Scientific Theories and Folk Theories

Absolutist theoreticians of illness assume the universal nature of the premises of their own Western scientific culture. These premises are generalised both within Western societies and to non-Western cultures. These theorists regard Western scientific medicine as a preconceived statement of the nature of illness and disease. They then use this to discredit lay identifications of particular illnesses by identifying a 'true' or 'essential' illness. This confuses the respective domains of scientific and folk explanation. It is the folk rationale that provides the identification of a particular event as an illness and leads to its presentation to official medical practitioners. If we then try to substitute *their* scientific rationale for the folk rationale that was responsible for the presentation of the condition in the first place, we are merely confusing domains of explanation. Frequently, this substitution is associated with a simplistic mind/body dualism. Folk illnesses are assumed to be without any biological basis if scientific medicine is unable to identify a unitary disease with the folk condition from its own paradigm. This mistakes the role of theories as classificatory practices. 'Scientific' theories are just one way of ordering phenomena. 'Folk' theories can be as logical and coherent, while attending to different aspects of events and producing a different classification.

Cavalier treatment of folk medical theories is often justified on practical grounds by reference to the alleged superiority of Western science. Clearly, germ theories of disease had a greater pragmatic value than miasmatic theories. But this value needs to be seen in the context of a collectivity in which the culture invoked by competent members positively emphasises well-being and regards illness as a failure of rationality. Illich's (1975, pp.122-50) historical analysis of death suggests that this is not an assumption that can be made lightly. Only in our own time has death become the ultimate form of consumer resistance. Before that it was regarded not as medical failure, a breach of rationality, but something that came in time to us all. At the end of a good life lies a good death, and this is something that is to be accepted with equanimity and not to be fought against. In the words of Brillat-Savarin's ninety-three-year-old great-aunt quoted by Illich (1975, p.150n), 'If you ever get to my age you will see that death becomes as necessary as sleep'.

Efficacy of medical treatment is not an absolute but a relative concept set in a cultural context, which enables its users to know what is to count as a successful outcome for the treatment given. The standards of success are not necessarily the same as those applied in any other context. As sociologists, however, our concern is not with the practical efficiency of folk concepts in promoting health by the standards of our own milieu. Our interest is not in the part that folk theories play in promoting biophysical well-being but in their contribution towards the maintenance of social order (social order in general, not any particular set of social arrangements). How do theories of illness contribute to the construction of the social world that is experienced as real by members of the society within which such theories are current? It is by such means that we shall come to understand the social action of society members in the light of those features of their experienced-as-real world to which they attend. Of course, this may ultimately have important practical consequences. If we wish to further a moral crusade in favour of our definition of well-being, then it is clearly vital to be able to articulate it with the theories of those whom we are trying to persuade. A variety of anthropologists have documented how scientific medicine is most likely to be accepted when its theories articulate with folk theories, or when it can empirically demonstrate successes in the light of the standards of rationality within the culture (see, *inter alia,* Erasmus, 1952; Gould, 1957; Press, 1969; Schwartz, 1969).

Traditionally, philosophers of science have drawn a sharp distinction between lay knowledge and scientific knowledge (Nagel, 1961). Most people's knowledge throughout the world is viewed as inconsistent, partially clear, somewhat irrational and not testable. In contrast, there is a special kind of knowledge called scientific knowledge that is disinterested, provisional, rational and coherent. Science deals in truth; laymen deal in error. Schutz (1962) adopts the same division in discussing the realities of everyday life and scientific theorising. He contrasts the natural lay attitude with its unquestioning acceptance that things are in order as they are with the systematic and reflexive scepticism of the scientist. Schutz is one of the first writers to take commonsense knowledge seriously, and much of his work is devoted to an analysis of its structures and operations. Even in his work, however, common sense remains a pale cousin to the diamond-bright mind of the scientist. But if we discount the romantic claims of science and examine its actual conduct, then two problems immediately become apparent.

First, scientists do not seem to theorise very much. Kuhn (1970) argues that most of the time scientists do not reflect upon the conditions of their work but merely investigate problems presented as 'obvious' under the auspices of the paradigm of inquiry to which they subscribe. Elliot (1974) reports from observation of laboratory scientists at their work something of the dependence of science on everyday life. Science depends upon commonsense for its starting problems, for the physical and social organisation of its work settings and for the judgements of observed events. The world in which the scientist works is an everyday world that is taken as given. It relies on the same everyday judgements of what is real and reasonable as does the everyday world of any other member of the science and commonsense encounters, namely that lay theories and mistaken the character of the province of meaning he purports to analyse as the scientific attitude. It may be better to describe it as a *theoretical* attitude, to which anyone can resort when their paradigm for explaining phenomena becomes inadequate, whether this is under the conditions of a Kuhnian scientific revolution or of Garfinkel's attempts to break down trust in the routine character of everyday life. This approach also has the merit of accounting for the second difficulty that any attempt to sustain a distinction between science and commonsense encounters, namely that lay theories and scientific theories have empirically identical structures.

This is brought out very clearly by Horton (1971). He observes that the activity of theorising is basically the search for unity underlying an apparent diversity; for simplicity underlying apparent complexity; for order underlying apparent disorder; for regularity underlying apparent anomaly. It is an attempt to account for the manifest nature of the commonsense world, in which routine existence takes place, in terms of a scheme linking a limited number of entities or forces by a limited number of general principles. This scheme is linked to everyday experience by a set of correspondence rules that translate events in the former into events in the latter. In the course of this enterprise it is found that theories provide a wider causal context for events than that provided by commonsense. Commonsense is primarily a knowledge of the here and now; theorising, particularly important when commonsense breaks down or is called into question, allows recourse to factors removed in time and space or reveals them behind the superficial taken-for-granted facade of everyday life. Horton cites the case of illness among the Kalabari. They recognise many different diseases and their specific herbal remedies. Ordinarily, illness is simply diagnosed and treated by the sufferer's kin or a folk doctor. But if it fails to respond to such treatment this everyday paradigm is called into doubt and a diviner may be called in to try to link the illness into a wider causal context. The level of the theory shifts according to the nature of the problems involved.

Theorising first disintegrates the objects given in the commonsense world into different aspects. These elements are then abstracted and recombined into a new context of cause and effect, which often seems to involve drawing analogies from the familiar to the unfamiliar. Just as the Tiv draw analogies from their lineages to the geography of their area, so Spencer drew an analogy from post-Darwinian biology to human society. This process has limitations of course, and resemblances may be only partial. It is also true that models may develop in such a way as to obscure the conditions of their original formulation.

I do not however share Horton's conclusions about the value of behaviourism, nor do I fully accept the second part of his account dealing with the differences between traditional African thought and Western science. Indeed, in this section he backs away from the radical implications of his own thought and casts far less of a sceptical eye than seems justified on the claims of Western science. It is not at all clear, for example, that scientific theories are readily and ruthlessly scrapped as soon as they become unsatisfactory, or that theoretical systems are not protected against attack by taboos erected by the intellectual policemen of a community. However, this paper is very important for our present argument in its demonstration of the fundamental continuity of the structures of theoretical thought.

If we accept this argument, then the sociologist must accord a similar epistemological status to all theories about the social and material worlds. This has a number of interesting consequences. First, it opens the door to a sociology of medical knowledge. Scientific medical thinking can become a topic for inquiry as much as can folk medical thinking. We can analyse the conditions of medical knowledge, the methods by which it is produced and justified and the contexts of its use. We have many accounts of medical practice but curiously little data on doing medicine. These points are elaborated in later chapters.

But before going on I want to underline a second consequence of treating all theories as epistemologically equal; that is, that all action under the auspices of some theory is entitled to be regarded as rational within the domain of that theory. The evaluation of conduct by reference to classical notions of rationality is a sensible procedure only if the conduct itself is intentionally ordered by reference to those standards. It may be relevant, as Garfinkel (1967, pp.279-81) notes, to scientific theorisers because the socially sanctioned procedural rules of recognising credible knowledge among the community of scientists are oriented by reference to classical rationality. This is not the case in everyday life. Lewis (1963) notes the limitations of the classical model of rationality in the case of seeking treatment for illness. He notes that the prevailing notion in this model - that the rational decision is the one that offers the maximum utility - depends on two assumptions: that the actor has accurate information, and that there is a series of events over which decisions are made rather than only one or a few. Lewis shows that these assumptions seldom hold true in practice but that nevertheless actors do proceed in a way that maximises their subjective utility in the light of the data available to them. In this context it is absurd to call their action non-rational. Scott (1968, pp.171-80) shows that the apparently random events of horse racing can be presented as rational in the light of the theorising of a race-goer. If we can come to take that theorising seriously, rather than merely seeking to substitute our own standards and discredit it, we can see that racing is as much a rational activity for the punter as philosophy is for the philosopher. If we insist on imposing our own standards, we merely disorganise and confuse a world that is in perfect order for its participants.

Treating all theories as epistemologically equal does not necessarily mean that we cannot talk about some theories as being better than others. We probably cannot say that one theory is truer or more valid, in any absolute sense, than any other: truth is seen as fundamentally social in origin; it is that which is accepted as true for that time and that place and has no necessary universal dimension. Nevertheless, we can say that some theories are more efficient than others. Erasmus (1952), for example, shows how Ecuadorian peasants came to accept the ability of Western doctors to cure yaws largely through their own empirical observation of the greater efficacy of their treatment. Preventive programmes, which depend upon a thorough appreciation of germ theories of disease, encountered much greater resistance. The methods prescribed by folk theories may be less effective in achieving the goals embedded in those theories but remain vulnerable to replacement by other more effective methods, generated within the community or imported from outside. This lack of effectiveness, however, does not entitle us to regard the theories as generally inferior. That depends on value judgements, like the moral desirability of reducing infantile death rates. Apart from this particular point of the efficacy of means in achieving ends, decisions between theories are moral decisions and the superiority of any one over any other is a matter of value judgements rather than scientific judgements.

It may be convenient at this point to state my own position. I have argued that all forms of theorising are, for the sociologist, equally valid ways of organising the world. They provide for the rationality of conduct under their auspices and allow actors to recognise and maintain the normal and routine character of everyday life and to identify possible troubles and formulate remedial courses of action. Descriptions of theories have an unavoidably problematic relation to particular courses of action. This is either because they are produced from accounts given when actors are invited to theorise about their actions (and this theory-in-theorising may not be the game as theory-in-action) or because the observer is obliged to try to induce from observed conduct the features to which actors are orienting their actions and to link these into a theory.

I conceive of social action as both produced and decoded, or made sense of, by drawing on theories. In particular, people draw on commonsense knowledge of social structures. This involves ideas about the nature of the society in which they are living and the social world that competent members of the society have to be able to show each other that they are living in if they are to be recognised as normal, rational, reasonable, etc. They contain ideas about the typical sorts of people and situations one is likely to meet and the ways of conducting oneself that are likely to be appropriate. These theories form a folk- or ethnosociology. They parallel those of traditional sociology, which is why that enterprise cannot account for social action but merely glosses it by substituting its own descriptions for those used by actors. The social and material worlds take on their meaning and significance only by virtue of interpretation in the light of these theories. Such interpretations may be limited, since neither the social nor the material world is infinitely plastic. However the significance of these limits still necessarily derives from the way actors interpret the world around them. 'Illnesses' are terms employed by sufferers, and those with whom they interact, to make sense of events in their lives. As I have suggested in this chapter, they cannot satisfactorily be regarded as either biological or behavioural essences. They are, rather, produced by using theories about the typical ways of experiencing one's own body or of observing the bodies of others and about the typical structures and functions that are found and the typical and atypical deviations that may arise. These theories provide socially sanctioned grounds for inquiring into the nature of an experience, identifying it (which may involve assigning a name or recognising that there is no name that can be assigned and launching a further inquiry), and justifying one's decisions about aetiology, diagnosis, therapy and prognosis. 'Illness behaviour' is the outcome of such processes.

4   Illness and Everyday Life

We have seen in earlier chapters something of the past tradition in studying illness and its social concomitants. I have tried to summarise the various treatments that have been accorded to this topic and to develop a set of arguments against them. In this chapter I turn to more positive proposals. I shall set out a model of illness based on the practical circumstances of everyday social life. Illness is depicted as a failure of rationality in particular kinds of settings ordered by particular kinds of cultural theories. The conceptual points made in this chapter are subsequently developed and illustrated by a re-analysis of various ethnographic accounts of illness and by a discussion of various methodological proposals that might bear on the themes elaborated here.

I have argued for a particular conception of the relationship between mind and body. I suggest that biological events occurring in human bodies are no more intrinsically meaningful than any other natural or social phenomena. They likewise need to be cognitively organised and interpreted before becoming relevant conditions for social action. This may of course include recognition of one's lack of comprehension and the need for inquiry as well as a positive identification of the phenomenon. Biological events may of course to some degree impose limits on the available possibilities for action, as in the case of paralysis, for example. However, for the socially competent actor, the sense and import of those limits is a cognitive phenomenon. (For the socially incompetent, like children, the mentally subnormal or the comatose, limits on action may be cognitively organised for them by others who are socially licensed, like parents, guardians, or attendants.) The limitations that paralysis imposes take on a meaning only in the context of the desires of the paralysed individual. The meaning of paralysis may be very different for a would-be Olympic athlete and a would-be novelist.

A sociological account of illness will require us to analyse the theories that individuals make use of in the context of disease. But since 'disease' is itself a culturally bound category, our enterprise will inevitably be distorted unless we can provide some alternative that respects folk categories. Taken thus, our study may include phenomena to which an ethnorubric of 'medicine' is not applied but which are subsumed under 'religion' or 'witchcraft'. Disease, then, is a change in an actor's state-of-being, which is seen as discontinuous with his everyday state-of-being. Moreover, as I argue later, it is treated as a special case of deviance, since in McHugh's (1970) terms, theoreticity or conscious responsibility is not invariably imputed to the sufferer. This change in state-of-being may have a readily identifiable biological parallel in the activity of a virus, a drug or some other biologically active agent. But the biological and the behavioural are logically independent.

A group's culture, particularly as embodied in its primary communicative device, its language, is, then, an especially important factor in our investigations. Language is the principal medium for the transmission of culturally acceptable theories about the material and social world and for their negotiation and validation in everyday encounters. In some measure this may be constrained by the material conditions of a group. It would be odd for a people who lacked access to body interiors to have an elaborated ethnoanatomy, for example. But this does not affect the central role of language in mediating everyday experience.

Before we can begin our investigation of the social nature of illness, however, a prior topic must be dealt with. And this is the nature of wellness. If we are to recognise illness, as with any other form of unusual and potentially deviant conduct, we need to be able to recognise wellness or normality. Illness and health form a contrasting pair so that we cannot recognise one without trading on our knowledge of the other. The nature of health, however, is less straightforward than might at first appear. We might propose that health was simply the absence of disease, for instance. But, if the relationship of illness and health is one of logical exclusion, as suggested above, then it follows that if health is the absence of illness, then illness is merely the absence of health and we find ourselves going round in ever-decreasing circles. Given the unobtrusiveness of what is normal, by virtue of its very normality, the unusual may be easier to identify. But it is recognisable *only* as a result of our trading on tacit and unexamined knowledge about normality.

There *have* been some attempts to provide non-circular definitions of health. A good example is that given in the charter of the World Health Organisation with the Utopian proclamation that 'health is a state of complete physical, mental and social well-being and not merely the absence of disease or infirmity'. As a proposition this is completely vacuous because we have no indication as to what might count as a state of complete well-being. Lewis notes how assessments of health and illness cannot be taken as absolutes but must depend upon encounters between doctors and patients:

> ... the physician must take the patient pretty much as supplying his own norm
> of total performance or behaviour, and proceed by rough and ready appraisal
> of whether there has been any departure from this, when due allowance has
> been made for the environment in which the patient is living. (Lewis, 1953,
> p.113)

Recognition of complete wellbeing still involves trading on unexamined commonsense conceptions of what counts as normal variation and what lies beyond that. For convenience, let us bracket together health, normality and ordinariness as terms that may be applied to a certain range of activities in certain settings, and deviance and illness as terms that may be applied to activities falling outside that range. I shall make certain distinctions between deviance and illness later in this chapter, but these are not important here.

Ordinariness as a Problem

(This section draws heavily on unpublished lecture notes by Harvey Sacks, particularly those for his lecture of 2 April 1970.)

Occasions of deviance or illness are special instances of the general case of observations that things are not as they should be. If we make a statement of the kind 'X is absent', like 'Smith has a fever' (i.e. an absence of normal temperature), the observation of absence must be discriminatory. That is to say, there is an infinite number of things that *might* have been present but we are orienting towards some finite and discrete collection. In this example, Smith's temperature *might* be anywhere between absolute zero and infinity, but we are orienting towards the collection of temperatures $98.4° F \pm 0.5° F$. To say that someone is deviant (ill), then, presupposes both some notion of what being normal (well) is and the relevance of affirming normality or calling attention to its absence.

Ordinariness is not an essential quality of acts but is produced by the interpersonal work of actors. Reports of social events, in conversation for example, are often less concerned with what actually happened than with demonstrating the ordinary character of events. This example is taken from an interview between myself and a physically disabled girl with a considerable orthopaedic deformity:

R.D.: Mmm What sort of things depress you?

Jill: Just simple everyday things, *just* have arguments with people and *your* parents and ... get bored with going to the same place and meeting the same people, *you know.* I just want to get away from it for a while.

While this is simply an illustration, I suggest that Jill's answer does show this general point. It is not a simple list of things that depress her but an attempt to demonstrate that, although disabled, she is essentially ordinary. I am not going to analyse this exhaustively, but merely call attention to the work that is being done by the italicised words and the way they appeal to the presumed level of background knowledge possessed by the by the hearer. 'You know' and its equivalents play a particularly crucial role in this process. Ordinariness, normality, health are the accomplishments of people working for and with each other to achieve mutual recognition. Like any other kind of work this requires knowledge, acquired through training and experience, resources and effort. Let us take these in turn.

How do people actually go about 'being ordinary'? At one level the answer is obvious. They do usual things in usual ways at usual times and in usual places. This does not mean simply that they are doing the same things as lots of other people, but that all the parties to a given situation are conducting themselves in the light of their knowledge of what ordinary people do in such situations. This involves two immediate issues: you have to know what anybody and everybody does ordinarily, and you have to be able to do it.

This knowledge of ordinariness is what Cicourel (1973) seems to have in mind in his discussion of 'commonsense knowledge of social structures', which I have analysed as 'members' social theories' (Dingwall, 1974, 1977). It is a body of knowledge about the typical sorts of persons and situations likely to be encountered and the relevant courses of action to adopt, that allows the recognition of what to count as normal conduct, and that allows its user to be recognised as a competent member of some collectivity by other members and, in turn, to recognise those others as competent members of that same collectivity. Some elements of this knowledge may he widely shared; others, more specialised and socially distributed. In the present instance, we are particularly interested in knowledge about the human body.

Birdwhistell (1973) discusses how people learn to manage their bodies in a fashion that members of their collectivity regard as competent. He points out that, while the human body is theoretically capable of a multitude of movements and postures, *in fact* the observable repertoire in fully competent collectivity members - normal adults - is quite limited. The infant is an amoral wriggler and babbler but comes to participate in a moral community of socially recognised vocalisations and body movements. Because we have an adequate independent coding system for speech in phonetic transcription systems, we can recognise speech learning in small babies. It is only the lack of an equivalent coding system for body management that prevents our discerning similar culture patterning in that sphere. Birdwhistell notes that psychiatric patients, for example, although apparently exhibiting bizarre postures, do not use any posture that is not part of the repertoire available within *their* culture. Their deviance lies in inappropriate situational performance or sequential ordering of movements. Birdwhistell records how differences in the performance of gender can be identified in this dimension: characteristically, men and women manage their bodies in a different fashion. I have also identified status differences, even without the need to use Birdwhistell's precise notational system. In my research on health visitors (Dingwall, 1974, 1977) I showed how body management could be a feature of discriminating 'professionals' from 'non-professionals'. For student health visitors, one element of achieving recognition as competent members of the occupation, with its claimed status as a profession, was the adoption of 'professional' body management. Body management, then, is not to be seen as an innate system: it is a social construct, which takes on significance through the interpretive work of competent culture members. On this point we part decisively from the ethologists.

This opens up a whole series of possibilities for the study of the physically disabled, to which we shall return in discussing the question of resources. Before this however I would like to illustrate the issue of health knowledge. We have noted that body management is to be seen as a voluntary process, deriving from a recognition of the socially sanctionable body forms available to members of any particular collectivity. I suggest that we can parallel this by an identification of some form of knowledge about normal body operations. On this point I do not want to press the issue of voluntary, even if routinely taken-for-granted, control, although I think we should treat this as an open question. *Pace* the remarkable achievements reported of Indian fakirs, I feel on firmer ground if I adopt the less radical position that biological processes carry on in a more or less autonomous fashion. We can then merely suggest that knowledge of normal operations is used by individuals to monitor the systems of their own bodies, and those of others, for changes which might have implications for future actions.

Unfortunately, there is something of a dearth of detailed empirical reports in this area. We know rather more about ethno-illness than we do about ethno-health. However, Schulman and Smith (1963) do offer us a useful account of the concept of 'health' among Spanish-speaking villagers in the American South-West. They show that health is a background feature of daily living and of a person's display of his essential normality - 'Healthy people are normal and normal people are healthy' (p.228). But health is always a situated concept. If someone is healthy they are healthy for the here-and-now, or perhaps 'until further notice'. Just as warranting one's claim to be considered a competent member of some collectivity by establishing one's normality is a continuous process, so too is the establishment of one's essential health. Health is related to the typical expectations of particular sorts of individuals. At one level characteristics of health are widely shared 'as common health denominators of adequately functioning community members'. Such common denominators include a high level of physical activity, a well-fleshed body and an absence of pain. But the interpretation of these is inevitably keyed to a typification of their subject. For example, the standards by which Anglo-Americans are judged are set against a conception of health that is different from that of the Spanish-speakers. Similarly, the conceptions of health in children and old people, while formally displaying these general properties, are tied to what is routinely expected of the young and the old. The standard of activity by which an old person's health is judged, for example, is one that relates to typical old people rather than to all villagers or to typical mature adults.

In addition to having access to the knowledge upon which members of some collectivity must draw to affirm their competence that they are normal, healthy or whatever actors must also have the resources to realise that knowledge in action. 'Resources' here is a fairly elastic term. It may just be a question of finance or material goods, but it can also include features of the body and its management. The physically disabled, for example, can be viewed as lacking a full repertoire of interactionally relevant resources. This, incidentally, allows us to dispose of the spurious cry that 'we are all handicapped'. Such self-delusion may be an interesting tactic but obscures the task of analysis. It might be true that if I was running over a hundred metres against the Olympic champion I would be 'handicapped'. It is absurd to suggest that either of us would be faced with a charge of interactional incompetence on the basis of the physical difference between us. One of the best illustrations of the conception of disability as a lack of relevant resources is Garfinkel's (1967) discussion of the transsexual Agnes. One can view her as a would-be ordinary woman attempting to live a normal life while being grossly disabled for that life.

In passing, we can also note how doing usual things also calls for us not to do unusual things. The collection of possible actions that count as normality is a finite one: some of the things disabled persons find it necessary to do, like paying conscious attention to excretion management in ulcerative colitis as described by Reif (1973) or adopting idiosyncratic gaits in comparison with the 'normal walking' described by Ryave and Schenkein (1974) and Wolff (1973), may fall outside this finite collection and merely reaffirm their deviance.

Being healthy, then, is not merely a matter of knowing how to display one's health, but also of having the resources to accomplish such a display. A lack of either may call the actor's status into question. But it is also important to note how the availability of resources is culturally organised. Knowledge about the body can, ultimately, be conveyed only through language, which draws attention to and sanctions appropriate and inappropriate models of being. The social world is possible only because of the availability of communication between one person and another out of which social order can be constructed. As Wittgenstein (1972, 1974) saw, language is the embodiment of a form of life, a way of living and of construing the world, and it is also the limit of the way of knowing the world. The possibilities of that form of life are the possibilities of the language that constitutes it. So, if we are trying to analyse the knowledge and resources that are available to members of some collectivity within the available form of life, we must attend to the possibilities of the language that constitutes that form of life, that collectivity.

The availability of suitable descriptions in a language is not, however, independent of the material circumstances of the collectivity. We have to take into account the mode of existence of the collectivity and the climatic and geographical conditions which may impose their own relevance as limiting conditions for members' actions. Hence it is hardly surprising that rice-growing Filipinos have numerous words for rice, Somali nomads have many words for camels, Sudanese herdsmen have many words for cattle and Eskimos have many words for snow. The ability to make fine discriminations on these subjects is important for the maintenance of collectivity members' well-being and way of life.

Similarly, the availability of language to describe the body is itself circumscribed by the technology available to members of a collectivity. Marsh and Laughlin (1956) describe the anatomical studies of the Aleutian Islanders. The Aleuts have developed an elaborate body of medical theory and practice based upon a detailed study of anatomy. Five sources for this knowledge are identified:

(i)   the Aleuts are almost exclusively dependent on hunting for their subsistence, which gives them a detailed knowledge of animal tissue, particularly in the light of their interest in utilising as much of the body as possible;

(ii)   Aleut doctors engage in detailed observation and experiment with both humans and other mammals, including,

(iii)   human dissection and

(iv)   comparative dissection of other mammals;

(v)   the mummification of distinguished individuals to defer decay and so retain the aid of the soul of the departed to the living.

Marsh and Laughlin present a list of several hundred anatomical terms collected from both lay and ethnoprofessional informants. They also note that the Aleuts recognise the processes of growth, such as the closure of the fontanelle and the hardening of soft bones, and most of the pulse spots. Treatments include a version of acupuncture, blood-letting, massage, manipulation, surgery, diet and rest. Apart from its therapeutic value, this knowledge was also used in wrestling and combat and the ritual dismemberment of fallen enemies, as well as in mummification.

We must however beware of ascribing some form of technological determinism. Admittedly, the Aleuts' material existence furnished them with the opportunity to engage in anatomical investigations, which I think we may take to be a necessary condition for the development of an elaborate lexicon. However this condition is not a sufficient one. Without the religious beliefs that permitted mummification and the dissection of available corpses, whether of enemies or of serfs, it would not have been possible to generalise confidently from animal to human. Thus if we compare the Aleuts and other Alaskan Eskimos with Arctic Sea coast Eskimos, we can see that, although the latter group are also a hunting people, their shamanistic explanations of illness give them no rationale for engaging in anatomical or other investigation. On the East coast, body disturbances are considered to have a spiritual origin and to require spiritual treatment. Marsh and Laughlin do not give an explicit description of Aleut theories of illness origins, but it seems to involve an ethnophysiology of 'bad airs' and 'bad blood' and a distinctive realm of ethnomedical theorising as opposed to a global appeal to spiritual or religious explanation.

We can illuminate this further by looking at other cultures with a direct prohibition against too close an interest in the body. Landar and Casagrande (1962), for example, recorded a fairly vague and limited anatomical vocabulary among Navaho Indian informants. The Navaho economy is pastoral, involving herding of sheep, goats and other livestock. Thus, the Navaho have the opportunity to acquire butchering experience and to use this as a source of inferences about human bodies. However, their interest in human corpses is limited by fear of ghosts and the desire to avoid imputations of witchcraft. Nor do they have any particular motive for risking inquiry, since illness is viewed as the product of cosmic disharmony brought about by sorcery or a breach of taboos rather than as the result of some biological disturbance.

In contrast, our own society permits ready access to the internal systems of the body, whether of the living or the dead. In part, this is clearly a function of technology. Without anaesthetics and antiseptics, X-rays and intubation, reliable access to the inner workings of the living body would be difficult. But it is equally a function of the changing nature of ideas about the human body. This is not merely a question of the availability of corpses for autopsy, although in Britain this did provoke public concern well into the nineteenth century as, for example, in the 1831 riots in Aberdeen when a mob of several thousand people set fire to the newly built Anatomical Theatre. The availability of corpses was little problem in Continental Europe however. Foucault (1973, p.125) is quite adamant that there was no shortage of suitable material in eighteenth-century France, while Waddington (1973, pp.220-1) notes the ample facilities for dissection and the support extended by the French government in the early part of the nineteenth century. Both Foucault and Waddington observe the critical role played by French doctors in medical developments: Foucault concentrates on the theoretical shift from a metaphysical to a rationalist conception of medicine; Waddington examines the structural changes in medical practice as a consequence of the expansion of health care facilities by the Revolutionary government. The modern hospital and the field that it offered for purposive-rational investigation was thus the consequence of both a cultural shift and a new political direction. This brings us back to my earlier discussion of Habermas's (1971, pp.81-122) analysis of the spread of purposive-rational thinking as a characteristic feature of capitalist societies. The economic transformations of the early nineteenth century are parallelled by intellectual transformations. It would be an error to ascribe to either a clearly determining role in relation to the other, but the interaction between material and intellectual factors led to their mutual elaboration and extension.

Such an interface of culture and technology has allowed us to develop an extensive and detailed vocabulary that makes possible elaborate and finely grained concepts of the body. This is not to deny that the degree of access to this vocabulary is socially distributed. Like the Aleuts, we have specialists in this domain of experience whose particular interests are going to require a more detailed vocabulary capable of finer distinctions than those needed by laymen. Nevertheless, the average member of our society has this whole lexicon potentially available and, although this is an empirical question, is likely to have a more extensive vocabulary directly at hand than, say, the average Navaho.

In their discussion of health maintenance among Quechua- and Spanish-speaking peasants in Peru, Fabrega and Manning (1972) note that bodily changes are experienced in a diffuse and heterogeneous fashion and can achieve a degree of uniformity only through linguistic activities. They propose that visible parts of the body and disturbances in them are more likely to achieve some degree of uniformity both within and between cultural groups, but that the less directly observable they are, the less standardisation there is likely to be and the more explanatory and diagnostic diversity one is likely to encounter. We can set their findings of heterogeneity in Quechua reports of disease and treatment alongside Stark's (1969) account of Quechua terms for visible parts of the body, which seem well defined and generally agreed, to suggest that this is indeed a plausible hypothesis. Further investigations might find it highly profitable to examine the question of whether visible injuries like fractures and lacerations fall into different folk categories than more amorphous diseases. It would be useful to know, for example, whether, in a culture where inner diseases are ascribed to spirit intervention and treated by appeals to those spirits, the same explanation extends to broken limbs in establishing both their origin and their treatment. I suspect that ascribed causality is likely to be continuous but that spiritual treatment is more likely to be complemented by some kind of direct physical intervention.

I have, then, set forth the kinds of knowledge and resources that are involved in any presentation of the actor as 'healthy'. I have suggested that the knowledge that competent members of any given collectivity draw on is necessarily constrained by the material circumstances of their collectivity. This should not be taken to mean that it is determined by those material factors. The transaction between ideas and material existence is two-way. I also noted that the ability of individuals to implement the requirements of this socially available knowledge in presenting themselves in interaction may be limited. These limits may reflect an impairment of the physical repertoire called for to sustain competent membership in the collectivity. Such an impairment may be due to a temporary or permanent absence or constraint of some bodily structure or function, for example a missing limb or a feverish disturbance of the biological systems of the body resulting from some pathogenic invasion. Other limited resources may be economic, intellectual or motivational. An individual may be unable to afford regular dental prophylaxis, to understand the need for excretion control or lack the will to renounce some addictive substance. All of these can impair the demonstration of one's essential 'health' as a normal and ordinary member of some collectivity where the background knowledge necessary to be accepted as a competent person provides for, in this instance, healthy dentition, excretion to be limited to certain segregated contexts and freedom from dependence on any pharmacologically active substance.

The question of motivation requires some further study. So far, I have been describing what is involved in presenting oneself as healthy. In order to move towards a discussion of illness, we need to recognise how presentation of oneself as a healthy individual is not merely an available possibility, but is also an enforceable one. The theories of social order that collectivity members draw on are not merely descriptive but are equally prescriptive. They specify not only what people and situations under the auspices of that collectivity *do* look like, but also what they *ought* to look like. Social orders are necessarily also moral orders. Social actors are moral agents.

Following arguments developed by Puccetti (1968) and by Blum and McHugh (1971), Voysey (1975) sets out an approach to this issue of moral and motivated conduct. She begins from the conditions under which the term 'person' may be successfully ascribed to some entity. She argues that the entity must satisfy two conditions: first, that it has an *intellectual* character, both having access to and being able to invoke some symbolic conceptual scheme, and secondly, that it has a *moral* character, so that its conceptual scheme has a place for moral symbols. The concept of a person is the concept of a moral agent to whose behaviour one can properly impute a moral character. Only persons can have motives ascribed to them: motives can be imputed successfully only to entities who can be assumed to know what they are doing and to know that there are such things as motives. As a converse to these requirements for ascribing personhood to an entity by reference to its intellectual and moral nature and the consequent regard for its conduct as motivated, we might add that to claim recognition as a person an entity must be able to demonstrate that it possesses these characteristics. This is a critical matter for everyday living, since only persons are eligible for full membership of most human collectivities. The consequences of complete or partial failure are a loss or denial of civil liberties. The constraints placed on groups like children, the old and the mentally ill reflect their inability to satisfy the above criteria. I shall discuss this point at more length in examining the relationship between deviance and normality.

However, this abstract formula needs to be expanded for analytic purposes. While it may make a general statement about the conditions for ascribing personhood, the particular occasions on which such an ascription is made will require a more particular formulation. In short, what is to count as recognisably intellectual and moral depends upon a variety of situational features. The ascription of personhood takes place within a social context whose features are constituted through interpretations drawn from a socially available stock of knowledge. Those entities recognised as persons achieve this by virtue of the interpretations placed on their conduct by others, generally recognised as persons. Such interpretations take place against a background of knowledge which it is assumed every 'person' shares. Both actor and observer are required to demonstrate their orientation to this knowledge if they are to be recognised as persons. In this light, personhood ascription is a particular case of membership ascription. It is the achievement of membership in the collectivity of persons.

This situational emphasis is important if we are to avoid creating a new absolutism. The issues of the intellectual and moral status of actors are not simple or clear-cut. One of the most frequently cited examples here is that of numerous North American Indian tribes which make no linguistic distinction between the term for 'person' and the term for 'member of the tribe'. This is not merely an anthropological curio. One might suggest that it indicates that, for these peoples, the universe of persons is coterminous with themselves. Others not of the tribe have a non-person status and as such cannot accept obligations or expect rights. Reflecting on our own society, it is not universally agreed that certain groups are to be regarded as persons: we have always been quick to identify indigenous populations in our colonies as 'primitives' or 'savages' and to deny them the status of persons. Similarly, there are those who will argue that blacks, football supporters or students are not fully human and are not therefore entitled to participate in the community of persons and to be eligible for membership of any of the various collectivities within that community. One of our future tasks as sociologists could well be the precise description and analysis of the situational conditions under which personhood may be ascribed or denied.

Morality is, then, viewed as situational. The nature of the morality reflects the nature of the situation. Douglas (1971) observes how public situations involve a lowest-common-denominator absolutist morality that is enforced by a variety of control agencies. This is presented as the only possible way of life and minimal public adherence is demanded as a condition for being recognised as a respectable, normal, healthy moral person. Surrounded by institutions of privacy, however, arenas exist in which private acts or beliefs may be expressed in the light of situational moralities, like the nudist camps described by Weinberg (1970). While such institutions limit the intervention of public control agencies, they also constrain the availability of alternative versions of everyday reality and thus assist the maintenance of the public order. There is something of a tension between the private and public spheres of life. Privacy may depend upon a public display of normality as Voysey (1975) argues. In her study of families with a disabled child, she suggests that the child constitutes a permanent charge of deviance against the family and invites the attention of control agencies. To defeat this charge, parents develop public accounts that display a conspicuous normality to control agents. Conversely, control agencies may, given their mandate to uphold public order, feel constrained to intervene in the private sphere to limit alternative possibilities of viewing everyday reality, whether through psychedelic drug use or political innovation. We can also note the tendencies towards the routinisation of consumption described by Young (1971). Young argues that the attempts of modern industry to render predictable the demand for its goods involve an increasing penetration of the private sphere of life in an attempt to control the available choice and to order the requirements of individual tastes. Against this can be set the occasions on which private spheres break out and have a lasting impact on the public. Political revolutions might be a good example. Even here however we should be careful not to overstate the case. Private realities are partial while public realities are global. When a private reality floods out it rarely produces a total reconstruction of the public but merely a partial reconstruction in its area of relevance. With the possible exception of China, no revolution has approached a total reconstruction of everyday reality. Much of the ordinary business of living is as ordinary as ever.

I am, then, suggesting that health should be seen as every bit as much a moral category as any other feature of everyday activity. For anyone to be recognised as socially competent, he needs to display his essential normality so far as is possible. By 'essential normality', I mean that, if a charge of deviance is made against some individual, he can point to relevant features of his life in an attempt to defeat the charge. Such charges may be made, in circumstances that I discuss below, but can be countered by an assertion that, notwithstanding appearances, the object of the charge is normal. Examples of this tactic can be found in Voysey (1975), where she analyses the accounts of family life given by parents of disabled children, and in Edgerton (1968), where he discusses the ways in which former patients of an institution for the mentally subnormal seek to counter the charge of incompetence as persons by appealing to certain features of their everyday lives, for example their work, family and social activities. The assertion of the moral nature of health is, however, difficult to illustrate except by reference to the moral nature of illness. I shall analyse this more fully in the next section, but a nice example of the way that the assertion of one's essential health may be enforceable on anyone claiming social competence can be found in the routine conversational opening 'How are you?'. This is almost invariably succeeded by an affirmation of health. Although such an affirmation may be followed by a specification of afflictions, these are presented as modifications to a state of essential health.

More generally, we might apply the kind of analysis set out by Dexter (1962, 1964) in his remarks on mental subnormality. He points out that the social discrimination against the stupid is based on the organisation of our society around individual intellectual skill regardless of the needs of the task in hand or the possibility of group working, which would allow each group to use the strengths and cover the weaknesses of its several members. Mental subnormality is a political problem by virtue of the failure of the stupid to manage their lives in accord with the demands of control agencies upholding the public morality. Similarly, illness is a political problem since ours is a society arranged on assumptions of health. This manifests itself in several ways. For example, one can suggest that there is an increasing premium on personal mobility for a whole range of everyday activities. Fagerhaugh's (1973) discussion of emphysema patients brings out clearly the problems that a restricted oxygen supply and consequent lack of energy give rise to in daily living. To some degree, time, money and energy can be traded off against each other, but a severe deficiency in one dislocates the pattern beyond the range of normal accommodations. Similarly, places of work and work processes are laid out in ways that cannot absorb any degree of disability. Paradoxically, the increasing influence of ergonomics (engineering furniture and machinery to fit the physical capacities of the average person) may circumscribe the possible range of acceptable variation even further. Illness is a general threat to the ability of individuals to participate in the processes of production and consumption upon which the economic order depends. I shall return to these issues in the latter part of this chapter.

Illness and Deviance

One of the more vigorous debates within medical sociology in recent years has been on the issue of whether illness is or is not deviance. On the one hand there are those like Freidson (1971) and Twaddle (1973) who argue that illness fits the general sociological framework of deviance and needs distinguishing from other forms of deviance only by reference to the control agencies that police it. On the other hand, Robinson (1971), for example, argues that, since anyone is likely to fall sick (even members of sickness control agencies), this cannot be seen as motivated in the same way as crime or sin. It is only where these overlap with illness, as in the case of venereal infection and its alleged origin in loose living, that it is reasonable to think of illness as deviance.

In my view much of the confusion has arisen from differences in the usage of the term 'deviance'. If we accept the argument of the preceding chapters that to be accepted as a competent member of some collectivity a person must display that he is ordinary, healthy and normal by the standards of fellow members of that collectivity, then it follows that any lapse is, in some sense, deviance. Deviance may be used as a term to apply to any violation of a public morality, which is of course likely to draw the attention of the relevant control agencies. Some writers, however, reserve 'deviance' solely for terms like 'crime' and 'sin', which are more properly sub-categories of a more general usage. These categories may be either singly or severally relevant on particular occasions and are ordered in a hierarchy of censure. We can then accept that illness, in general, is not recognised as particularly reprehensible. On certain occasions, however, it may overlap with sin or crime, which carry more moral stigma. In these instances the condition derives its moral weight from the ascription of greatest severity. In this account, then, I prefer to regard 'deviance' as a cover term for a set including 'crime', 'sin' and 'illness' and all occasions when public order is breached, rather than counterposing it as motivated action against illness as unmotivated action.

This view follows McHugh's (1970) account of commonsense ascriptions of deviance. I argued, in my earlier consideration of Freidson's work, that the study of deviance needed to begin from its ascription in everyday settings. McHugh suggests that such ascription depends upon the view that potential ascribers take of the conventionality and theoreticity of some act that is presented to them. In these terms conventional behaviour is behaviour that the observer, whom we assume to be a competent member of some collectivity under whose auspices the behaviour is purporting to take place, considers might have taken place in some other fashion. (Although I can see McHugh's reasons for using 'conventional behaviour' at this point, I think his argument would have been clearer if he had described it as 'non-conventional' since we are dealing here with behaviour that is out of line with the relevant conventions of some setting. In order to avoid further confusion I have followed his usage, but the reader may find it helpful to reverse the polarities on these terms.)

Deviance is not, then, inevitable behaviour. It is identified in the light of possibilities for ordinary conduct, which it is presumed any competent collectivity member could discern in that situation. Deviance involves not merely not following some rule, but also the observer's ability to conceive of that rule being followable in the situation in which it was not followed. Since deviance ascription follows interpretive work by an observer, it does not involve labelling or tagging the behaviour as deviant, but rather levelling a charge of deviance. This recalls the view of Engel (1960), which I cited earlier, that the identification of a condition as illness depended upon an initial complaint, either by the sufferer or by others. McHugh's account tends to imply that charges may be levelled only by others, but clearly we may also find self-indictment, as in confession or self-criticism. The labelling of conduct as deviant is an epiphenomenon of this charge and of subsequent attempts to defeat it. The possibility of defeating the charge depends upon the success of appeals to some battery of possible grounds for refuting the accusation. This may involve either self-defence, by an actor trying to refute an observer's accusation, or reassurance, by an observer trying to refute that actor's self-accusation. I have already touched on this point in my discussion of the way Voysey's families attempted to defeat charges of deviance by pointing to the underlying, essential normality of their situation, the model nature of their family life. These responses, justifications, excuses and rationalisations can form failure conditions for normal conduct, specifying the circumstances under which *any* competent person might be unable to act normally. They allow the actor to present the deviant behaviour as inevitable and the observer may accept it as such. Deviance is a failure to act in an explicable and predictable fashion when no failure conditions are available to defeat the charge of deviance.

The second element that McHugh identifies relates to an actor's theoreticity, that is to say the extent to which he is taken to be aware of what he is doing. A theoretic actor is assumed to know what the relevant conduct is in any given situation and to intend his action in the light of this knowledge. Deviance is thus a knowing and wilful inattention to the correct behaviour.

Deviance ascription is a two-stage process. In the first, the observer evaluates the conventionality of the behaviour to determine whether it is unnecessary or whether there are possible grounds available to support it. This is the *prima facie* basis of a charge of deviance. The actor may be able to defeat this charge by pointing to reasons for his action that the observer had not foreseen. As I noted above, in certain cases actor and observer may be one and the same person. The actor may assess the conventionality of his own actual or intended conduct and the possible failure conditions surrounding it. For a charge of deviance to stick the actor must also be seen as a theoretic being who can be presumed to know what he is doing and be held responsible for his actions. Children, for example, are not usually treated as theoretic actors and may legitimately escape charges of deviance since they cannot be held responsible. It is important to note the way this parallels my earlier discussion of what it takes to be a moral person, a competent member of some collectivity. In this I presented individual actors as constrained to display their intellectual knowledge of the way of life under the auspices of that collectivity by being able to produce behaviour acceptable to other members of the collectivity and to display their moral sense so that this behaviour can be seen as intentional action by observers. Deviance and ordinariness are two sides of the same coin and are no more separable than the obverse and the reverse of that coin.

Conventionality and theoreticity may be combined in varying degrees with varying consequences. McHugh investigates the possible interpretations of observable false statements: a tactful remark may be regarded as non-conventional since it is required by considerations of politeness; a 'tall story' may be treated as an exercise of the imagination and the actor not regarded as theoretic; a paranoid delusion may be regarded as a conventional act by a non-theoretic actor, requiring therapy; a lie may be regarded as both conventional and theoretic, without excusing conditions and with intent, and may lead to punishment.

In his account McHugh shares the general neglect of physical illness, although he presents it as encompassing social deviance generally, including 'crime', 'sin' and 'mental illness'. I think, however, we can see how this might come under the model. The healthy person is seen as someone who is capable of pursuing relevant courses of action in the situations he encounters in everyday life within the orbit of the collectivities of which he claims membership. This implies not merely that he can be seen to do the right things but also that it can be reasonably inferred that he knows what he is doing. We may be able to train chimpanzees to have tea parties. but we do not readily ascribe to them the knowledge that what they are doing is 'having a tea party'. In this version, of course, health is inextricably tied up with other terms like ordinariness and normality. Illness is a particular form of failure at everyday life.

Illness is behaviour that is conventional and is, in this sense, clearly deviance. It is not in accord with what is to be reasonably expected, so that the ill person is someone who might have behaved otherwise but has failed to do so. A person who appears with red spots covering his face is *prima facie* failing to behave in a manner that is to be expected. He may be able to defeat this charge in a number of ways, for instance by suggesting that he has been made up in this fashion to appear as a patient in a television serial, or that he is *en route* to a fancy-dress party. If such grounds are not available then the charge of deviance may be pressed. At this point the theoretic status of the actor comes into play. To what degree can the ill person be held responsible for his condition? Some writers, notably Parsons (1951), have suggested that illness is by definition a form of deviance for which the sufferer cannot be held responsible. This is, however, now generally accepted to be an erroneous view. As Freidson (1971) shows, in summarising the debate, imputed responsibility is important for understanding the social consequences of illness. However Freidson does fall into the error of taking over medical diseases as a way of analysing the imputation of responsibility. The point here is that the same medical disease may be variously treated in accord with lay theories of causality and responsibility. If we take the instance of the common cold, lay theorising occasionally imputes a causal connection between wet feet and a cold. Now consider two possible, fictitious, case histories. Case A is a man who has got his feet wet rescuing a dog from a river some miles from his home. He returns home, changes his socks without delay and develops a cold some days later. Case B is a man who has got his feet wet during a rainstorm while shopping, sits around in his wet socks on returning home and develops a cold. Although both doctors and laymen might arrive at an identical diagnosis, the social consequences are likely to be quite different. Where both conventionality and theoreticity are ascribed in Case B, the consequences are likely to be punitive, while in Case A where the person cannot be held responsible for not changing his socks immediately, the emphasis is more likely to be therapeutic.

On the other hand, imputations of theoreticity may structure proposed aetiologies. A good example of this might be migraine, where moral evaluations of the normality of a person's life can shape the proposed causes. Thus, migraine may be imputed to women because they work or because they are staying at home, because they are married or because they are not married, because they have children or because they do not have children. We might find that a woman who worked as a night club dancer would have her migraine attributed to her employment while a woman doctor would have hers attributed to some metabolic disturbance. Since the general theoretic status of women seems to be regarded as more questionable than that of men, they may be particularly exposed to the influence of such imputations in accounting for disturbances in their physical state. It is a common feature of lay parlance to speak of women as more fanciful, irrational, irresponsible or whatever than men. The effect may be that physical pain or discomfort may be dismissed or played down since the complainant is not regarded as sufficiently responsible for her own actions to be taken seriously. This interplay between theoreticity and imputed aetiology can also be seen in the activities of groups of sufferers from some categories of illness where theoreticity may be implied to defeat this charge. Migraine sufferers tend to promote biochemical explanations of their disorder; associations of families with a schizophrenic member seek to discount explanations in terms of family disorder; and infertile persons argue that their inability to reproduce is due to *force majeure* rather than selfishness or sexual aberrance. Here we come back to my earlier suggestion about a hierarchy of censure. If we conceive of 'deviance' as a generic cover term for all categories of breaches of social order, then we may still allow that, within this sphere of conventional behaviour, there may be a number of categories distinguished by the degree of theoreticity that is imputed. It does appear that, the more an actor is held responsible, the more his condition will be regarded as intentionally provoked and deserving punishment rather than therapy. Illness is marked by a relatively low degree of theoreticity, but it may overlap with categories with a higher degree of theoreticity which set the tone for its treatment. Thus venereal disease may be counted as both illness and sin. The boundaries of the conditions for which responsibility is imputed do not necessarily correspond to the boundaries that doctors set on illness. In the case of the military, cowardice may be widely imputed where there is a possibility of self-inflicted injury or disease being used to avoid active service. The response may be punishment rather than therapy.

Much also depends on the status of the actor. It is unlikely that children would have responsibility imputed since they are not commonsensically regarded as theoretic actors. This, of course, does not mean that the parents might not have responsibility for their child's condition imputed to them as proxy theoretic actors for the child. If a child was afflicted by polio today, for example, the child would probably not be held responsible, but its parents might well be since it can be argued that they ought to have had the child vaccinated. Imputations of theoreticity shift over time. Army physicians seem to have been much readier to exempt soldiers from responsibility in the Second World War than in the First. Battlefield deserters could be identified as neurotic, not knowing what they were doing, and hence not responsible, rather than as cowards, knowing and responsible, and could face therapy rather than a firing squad. Ariès (1973) reminds us, in his classic account of the changing meaning of childhood, that the denial of theoreticity to children is of comparatively modern origin. In earlier times, children were likely to be treated as being as responsible for their acts as adults. Indeed, one can plausibly argue that one of the distinctive features of our modern world is the commonsensical withdrawal of theoreticity from increasing numbers of people. Children, lunatics, the aged, the alcoholic and the poor are all treated as if they are not to be held responsible for their own behaviour. It is entirely possible that this obscures more than it illuminates our understanding of social action that our public morality finds problematic.

In general, however, illness is not deviance for which theoreticity is ascribed. Indeed the phrase that often designates the withdrawal of theoreticity from a set of behaviours - the 'medicalisation of deviance' - gives tacit recognition to this point. Nevertheless, illness is no less of a problem to the public moral order than any other form of deviance. Health, as I have noted, is a moral phenomenon. Alternative states are threats to the public morality enforced by control agencies. They present alternative possibilities of being-in-the-world, and the availability of these options must necessarily be restricted if public order is to be maintained.

A persistent theme of this book has been that there are no illnesses or diseases in nature. Illness is the outcome of human classificatory activity. It is moreover a deeply moral activity, since health is identified as desirable and illness as undesirable. Sedgwick (1972) expands upon this point in his discussion of Dubos (1959). He notes that nature is morally organised by man in reflection to his anthropocentric self-interest. The blight on potatoes is a human invention, since we choose to cultivate the potato rather than the parasite; otherwise there would be no 'blight' but merely the necessary feedstuff for the parasite-crop. Viruses, fractures and malignancies similarly derive their import from human selection and ordering. In a somewhat purple phrase, Sedgwick sums up this argument: 'The fracture of a septuagenarian's femur has, within the world of nature, no more significance than the snapping of an autumn leaf from its twig'. 'Illness' and 'disease' are evaluative terms applied by man to natural circumstances that precipitate the death (or, more generally, prevent what he chooses to regard as adequate functioning) of a limited number of species: man himself, certain selected livestock and plant varieties grown for his use or pleasure. Control agencies, which include medicine, veterinary science and applied botany, operate around these to defend man's interests. Each of these operates under its own moral code, so that although euthanasia and eugenic breeding are not generally regarded as acceptable practices for humans, they are freely employed among animals and plants. Plant species in which we are interested can have diseases, like Dutch Elm Disease or mildew, but where we are not interested botanists merely report competition between species. Lay theories frequently subscribe to a black-and-white vision of the universe with the 'good germs' lining up alongside man to do battle with the 'bad germs'. In practice, of course, things are not that simple. It can be very difficult to decide whose side the germs are on. If we think of the so-called 'side effects' of drugs we can see how misleading words can be. 'Side effects', of course, merely refers to those effects that are not the desired central effect of the drug. The magic bullet may strike home but leaves its marks along the way. In fact side effects are as integral to the operation of the drug as the supposed therapeutic effect and can no more be disregarded than the passengers for Dundee who are occupying all the seats on a train we are taking for Edinburgh.

The morality in which health and illness are contained is defended, like other aspects of public morality, by a variety of control agencies. The defence of health is, however, a particularly tricky issue. Since theoreticity is not commonly ascribed to the sick, control agencies cannot generally depend upon explicitly punitive measures. Sickness may invite a certain amount of disapproval since the sufferer is unable to perform competently in the collectivities of which he is a member, like his family or his local community. It may involve inconveniences for the sufferer in its inhibitions on his economic and social activities. At the same time, it can entitle the sufferer to retire to his bed and demand economic and social support from others. Obviously the cost-benefit calculations involved are individual ones, hut there are also collective interests involved. Even the most Utopian community is going to depend upon some degree of productive activity, and if too many people act sick then the level of activity may be depressed below that necessary for the survival of the community. If public order is to persist then it is necessary to limit the attractiveness of alternative moralities. The process involved here is what we might call the 'privatisation of deviance'. In this account I want to analyse two particular elements: first, the formulation of deviance as trouble-in-the-family and, secondly, the development of institutions for its containment.

Illness and Family Life

Harvey Sacks has observed that it is a characteristic feature of social life that troubles are formulated as *someone's* troubles. Events, generally, are observed and reported as events-in-people's-lives; hence the importance of 'human interest' angles in media stories. An aeroplane crash does not just happen, it happens to some set of individuals and is an incident in their lives. Deviance is no different. It is deviance-in-some-people's-lives. A particularly common way of formulating such trouble is as 'trouble-in-the-family' which reflects the privatised nature of family life. Troubles in the family are their problem, not ours. The relevance of the problem is limited (to people in some particular membership category) by this device of assigning ownership of the relevant events. This forms a defence for us all against being overwhelmed by all the troubles in the world and effectively insulates the public as a whole from concern. However, this defence can be overturned through an attempt to formulate a problem as, say, 'trouble in *any* family' rather than as 'trouble-in-a-family'. People can then become personally involved on a massive scale since the trouble is seen as available and threatening to any and every family.

Illness is a good example of this process. Parsons and Fox (1952, p.37n) comment that the sick, unlike other deviants, are prevented from forming a solidary sub-culture, an alternative moral community. They attribute this to the intrinsic nature of sickness. However, I suggest that it is better explained by reference to the privatisation of sickness. Sickness is a trouble-in-someone's-life - the sufferer's. It disrupts his participation in those collectivities in which he holds membership. Most of these collectivities fall into the public domain where public morality can be enforced by control agencies. Since this morality has an absolutist character, the possible tolerance of deviance is rather limited. The deviant will consequently tend to be extruded from public life into spheres where his deviance is less threatening. These refuges from public life constitute the domain of the private. They are contained by the public sphere and partially insulated from it, offering time out from its absolutist demands. The family is often presented as a key institution in this respect (e.g. Berger and Kellner, 1964), but there is clearly a whole variety of such private worlds with their own reality-building, as Weinberg (1970) shows in his account of nudist camps, for example, or Warren (1974) describes in her account of gay communities in California. However, in most contexts, the family is arguably the commonest and most readily available private institution. Consequently, if illness is seen as trouble-in-the-family it can readily be insulated from public concern and the threat from individual deviance to public order can be countered. Consider in this light the difficulties that attend being sick while living alone, or the demands that it is felt can legitimately be made on family members at a time of sickness. It is, for example, quite acceptable to ask close kin to travel long distances, to suggest they move closer to the sufferer and generally rearrange their life to accommodate a sick family member. Sudnow (1967) shows how death is similarly organised as a family trouble in which close kin are expected to be most directly involved.

Parenthetically, illness also shows up the power of formulating trouble as trouble-in-any-family. A good example is the polio epidemic prior to the development of successful vaccines. Charitable organisations succeeded in presenting this as a random attacker that could visit even the most respectable of homes with tragedy. Indeed it seems that the most moral of citizens, the American bourgeoisie, were precisely the most likely victims since their children had no opportunity to acquire natural immunity. Polio charities attracted huge inflows of money for research and therapy. In the 1964 Aberdeen typhoid outbreak, the public health authorities presented the bacillus as a random attacker which threatened anybody and everybody and made a marked impact on the living standards of the whole city. Despite the diversion of resources to cope with the outbreak, the public health statistics showed no overall deterioration, and unparalleled standards of hygiene were maintained in food-handling and processing and in public conveniences. However, not every illness can be so treated. It seems that only non-theoretic conditions can be reformulated in this way. Members of afflicted families do not thereby find their sense of their essential normality threatened, as Davis

(1963, p.164) suggests in his discussion of the families of polio victims. They must also be perceived as representing a genuine threat. The common cold affects people fairly randomly, but since it is seen as trivial in its consequences we do not find mass concern. Whoever heard of Action for the Common Cold? Where an illness is likely to involve theoreticity being imputed to the family as a whole it may be difficult to turn it into a threat to *any* family. Thus, we have a rather lukewarm public response to many conditions where heredity is thought to be implicated, like Down's Syndrome, or where the family as a whole may be blamed, like mental illness. There is no interest in voluntary fund-raising for research in gonorrhoea, which is now one of the commonest infectious diseases and for which it would be technically relatively simple to develop an effective vaccine. Apart from the 'sin' dimension of venereal diseases, the ability of the family to absorb them is limited by the difficulty of reconciling them with the public principle of exclusive mutual sexual access between husband and wife upon which families are supposedly founded. Terminal illness may present rather similar problems in its intimation of the mortality of members in contrast to the immortality of institutions.

But against these tendencies towards the privatisation of illness needs to be set a long-term trend towards the diminution of areas of privacy. Compare family life in any modern society today with a century ago. There are two key elements at work here: the social relations within the family and the relations between the family and its environment. Both have been radically changed under the impact of urbanisation and changing patterns of economic organisation into large-scale state or private capitalism.

The decline of the extended family seems generally acknowledged. As a consequence, an area of autonomy from public life has diminished. The detailed scrutiny by kinfolk over the daily lives of other family members has been replaced by scrutiny from public control agents. Not infrequently this may well be a less oppressive experience for the individuals involved since the public morality may be a more permissive, lowest-common-denominator one and the surveillance may be far more haphazard. Against this may be far more enforceable uniformity in the practice of family life. While tolerance of unmarried couples or homosexual partners living together may have increased, the range of possible expressions may well have diminished. It is hard to imagine the continued existence of conspicuously eccentric households like those of Bertrand Russell or Augustus John in our own day. The demand for recognition of homosexual marriage may be a particularly telling example. We are not presented with some radical alternative pattern of living but merely an attempt to reformulate a relationship under the auspices of a well accepted public morality and to model homosexual living on a traditionally enforced heterosexual pattern. The process of substituting public for private morality has involved four principal elements.

First, we have the cult of domesticity. Lasch (1975) presents this as an integral part of the nineteenth-century religion of health. It is one element of the general attack on pre-industrial customs and the attempts to remodel the lives of the working classes by the forces of organised virtue. Industrial and social discipline were to be established upon a devastation of the collective forms of life that dominated traditional societies. The theorists of the new capitalism advocated a wholly individualistic form of social life. In the light of the rapid economic and technical changes of the period this was a view that would promote the interests of those with a stake in this modernisation'. The traditional forms of collective life stood in the way of 'progress'. Yet if they were swept aside, then so was their capacity for maintaining social discipline. Numerous replacements were offered. The traditional holidays and ceremonies were superseded by the sanitised festivals of Methodism. Workers were herded into factories governed by legalistic rule-books. The cult of domesticity elevated the enclave of the family as an isolated and insular retreat from the temptations of collective resistance to the economic and social changes. This is a process that is still going on throughout the underdeveloped world as peasants and slum-dwellers learn the requirements of factory discipline. Lasch notes the key role of the medical profession in all this. He presents them as the ministers of a new absolutist religion in the forefront of attempts to control the physical and mental welfare of the lower orders.

In the wake of this ideological change comes the second factor, the assumption by the State of tasks that had been carried out by the family, such as the day care of children and schooling. As Gilbert (1966) shows in his work on the origins of the British Welfare State, increased public intervention in family life was motivated by nationalist concerns about military and commercial weakness. Under the conditions of late nineteenth-century capitalism, families were failing to produce sufficient numbers of fit and well-educated workers and soldiers. The State was also threatened by subversion as the industrial, urban working class began to create its own organs of collective expression. The cult of domesticity was failing to produce the goods. The remedies adopted were twofold: certain tasks were taken over directly by the State, most notably education and, later, the care of the sick; secondly, State agents began to police the standards of home life, acquiring rights of entry, inspection and compulsion. Examples here would include sanitary inspection, health visiting, building inspection and the like. These interventions have obviously had real individual and social benefits - people do live longer and healthier lives, houses rarely blow up or fall down and children are less frequently assaulted or ill-nourished. On the other hand, such measures have reduced the area of privacy in everyday living.

Thirdly, we have the increasing importance of large corporations, whether privately or publicly owned. Watson (1964) argues that these depend increasingly on impersonal spiralist promotion systems. Employees are siphoned off, via the formal educational system, from their communities of origin and despatched as, where and when their talents are required. The social mobility of promotion is almost always associated with geographical mobility (hence the term 'spiralist'). In order to foster such mobility and to tie employees more closely to their employer, many of these corporations consciously attempt to limit the local connections of their employees. The consequences are an attenuation of kinship links and a tendency towards nuclearisation of family life.

Finally, we have the impact of social planning. Lefebvre (1971, p.122) notes that the inhabitant of the modern city is living in an environment that is fixed for him by the activities of public control agents. Their influence may be quite direct, in the case of those who live in public housing, or rather indirect, in the case of those living in private housing, which is nevertheless circumscribed by building regulations. Both are equally exposed to the vagaries of public transport systems and publicly regulated building for state or commercial purposes. Towns are no longer the creations of communal individuality but are planned entities imposed on their inhabitants. I think however that Lefebvre exaggerates the freedom of past ages in his rather general romanticisation of the past. Very few would have had the control over their dwelling that he implies, being obliged to rely on the taste of their landlord or of speculative builders. Although here, as with the extended family, we can see something of a plurality of definitions against the homogeneity of the contemporary situation. There is, nevertheless, a genuine point to be made about the degree to which the environment of family life is fixed or free and the possible definitions of family existence that are available.

These all reflect increasing constraints on the capacity of families to absorb any form of deviance, such as illness. The family with a sick member may be unable to travel lightly enough for spiralism, or to absorb its sick member into housing inflexibly planned for one particular pattern of family living. Everyday life in the modern city is designed around the abilities of the fit or of those who can purchase prosthetic substitutes. In her study of emphysema patients, for instance, Fagerhaugh (1973) shows how urban mobility is a matter of trading between time, energy and money. A deficit of one element, in this case energy, can be remedied only by a substitution of others. Family life involves similar trading. As an area of privacy - of timeout from working - it can nevertheless be sustained only by public activity. Family life may involve opportunity costs in working life because some benefits, such as increased leisure, have to be traded off against others, such as earning sufficient wages to support the quality of leisure activities. In particular, maintaining the quality of private life may entail increasing costs in purchasing insulation from public life, and attempts to manage the consumption of private goods and activities may increase the costs of a socially acceptable style of living. The necessary investment can prove too great a burden for the traditional division of household labour into a wage earner and a house-manager. Women may have been increasingly freed from home tasks by the State's development of rationalised child supervision and management agencies, but they now come under increasing pressures to engage in productive labour as wage-earners. This is not to deny the satisfactions and benefits that may accrue to the individuals involved, but there are certain consequences, which tend to fuel the processes at work here.

If we postulate a more or less constant proportion of GNP accruing to wages, then an increase in the labour force necessarily drives down the average level of real wages. Incomes accruing to a single party may become inadequate to maintain a household. Consequently, pressures on non-wage-earners in a household are increased and more people are likely to be drawn into the work force, accentuating the depression in real wages. Thus, it may increasingly be the case that two-person participation in the work force is a condition of family life. Something like this may well be behind the continuing fall in the birth rate. Yet the scheduling demands of a household with its two principals working are almost inevitably going to constrict the opportunities for privacy. To maintain any privacy in family life at all, tasks may have to be extruded from this sphere. In particular, the potential for containing deviance is severely reduced. Two possibilities exist: the redefinition of deviance, as in the case of gay rights movements, or the creation of new institutionalised areas of privacy under the control of public order agents, with the development of prisons, asylums, old people's homes and hospitals.

Before moving to a concluding analysis of hospital life, I want to add one or two comments on this section. First, I have not said anything about the everyday life of the rich or the famous. This requires a separate investigation which I cannot really pursue here. Briefly, one can suggest that certain people in our society are licensed to live 'epic lives'. Their everyday doings are a matter of public interest. It is only the Henry Kissingers of this world who have the contents of their dustbins stolen, listed and published in the press. Only royal families, presidents and the like have regular statements issued on their illnesses. The celebrity's life is intensely public; at the same time, it is only loosely controlled. Epic lives are not to be lived by the same standards as those of ordinary mortals. Secondly, the preceding analysis is not intentionally written as a moral critique. The obverse of the waning of privacy in everyday life and the limitations on the possibilities of individual deviance or dissent is a dramatic improvement in the quality of material life for many people and of enhanced opportunities for self-development, especially for women. Moral judgements on the balance of advantage are for the reader to make. Thirdly, the section should not be read as expressing economic determinism, although much of it borrows economic phraseology. Economics describes the outcomes of a series of individual judgements. Those judgements hang on the same kind of interpretive processes that I have emphasised throughout this book. The significance of material conditions for social action is the outcome of acts of recognition, formulation and description. Finally, where I have allowed myself to speculate about future events this is subject to the usual *ceteris paribus* assumption. To take an example, I have assumed that the net share of GNP accruing to wages will remain roughly constant. It may, of course, increase or diminish, with different effect on the material conditions that are available for social interpretation.

The Institutionalisation of Illness

My final theme in this chapter is a brief investigation of the role of the hospital as an institution for deviance control. It is not merely fanciful to regard the modern hospital and the prisons of the Spanish Inquisition as institutions of the same general type. They are, after all, both places into which people disappear from everyday life, some suddenly and some after prolonged investigation, and from which only a proportion ever emerge alive. Inside, bizarre and painful manipulations are performed on the victims' bodies by people who are honourable and respected members of a society and who are firmly convinced that these procedures are for the victims' own good. The workings of such 'total organisations', to borrow Goffman's (1968) term, are impervious to general public review. They form institutionalised zones of privacy within which public control agents can perform their mandate of containing social deviance and dissent.

The development of the hospital inverts our account of the development of modern family life. Among those families with the resources to sustain privacy, hospitalisation was resisted longest. Its encroachment began with the poor, whose dwellings and income fixed an environment in which the burden of non-productive family members could not be sustained for any appreciable length of time. By and large, hospitals were places where the poor went to die once their resources for sustaining private existence were exhausted. As such they were not particularly desirable places and on the whole probably did more harm than good through cross-infection and their general insanitary conditions. Of course, these conditions may well simply reflect those in the homes of many patients. However the hold of the principle of less eligibility, that those not productively employed should be clearly worse off than those in employment, over the State or charitable authorities who were responsible for theme institutions also played its part in depressing conditions. Treatment was provided either by doctors in training through experimentation at the voluntary hospitals or by the doctor willing to work for the lowest salary in Poor Law hospitals.

The general acceptance of hospitalisation by all classes of society is a phenomenon of the last thirty to forty years. Effective surgical intervention was available from the early years of the present century with the development and spread of anaesthetic and antiseptic techniques. Yet, for the most part, those who could offer the facilities for surgery at home still had operations performed there. To some measure this was a function of the available technology: surgery was a portable craft that could be performed anywhere a doctor could set up his kit; patients did not need to be brought to a specialised location with specialised resources available. But we cannot say that the state of the available technology determined the form of practice. That was a reflection of the ideas current at the time, which could he freely applied to the available environment. Nowadays, home surgery is not an available option except for the extravagantly rich. But at the time we are discussing, the doctors did have available the option of insisting that patients come to them. They chose not to take it up.

Effective medical intervention is an even more recent event. This really goes back no further than the Second World War, when antibiotics became generally available. Previously little could he offered other than skilled nursing, although an understanding of the transmission of disease had led to the development of sanatoria for the isolation and containment of contagious infection.

During the early years of this century there was a gradual development of private accommodation in hospitals for the use of middle-class patients, but this was still relatively insignificant in comparison with the number of public beds. Private medicine was practised either in the patient's home or in the aptly named 'nursing homes', which consciously attempted to reproduce the familiar environment of their patients, offering individual accommodation, highly personalised treatment and a wide choice of dietary regime and general diversions. The small size of the genuinely private sector in the hospitals taken over by the National Health Service can still be seen today. On this argument the expansion in demand for hospital beds since the creation of the NHS represents not merely the removal of financial disincentives but also a longer-term shift in the ability of the members of other social institutions, like the family, to accept a certain measure of illness or physical incapacity in other members. Increasing demand for hospital services is, after all, not exclusively a property of socialised health care systems. We should note, too, the attempts to make hospitals more home-like in the provision within them of more middle-class environments, enhanced standards of privacy, more varied diets, more scope for personal choice in diversionary activities and so on.

Nevertheless, hospitals tend to remain insulated from the society at large. These are, of course, matters of degree. The more patients' conduct is regarded as conventional and non-theoretic, the more insulated the institutions become. Hospitals for the mentally deviant, the subnormal and the lunatic are set in country areas or quasi-country. In part, of course, these are a residuum of earlier generations. Yet even here we are substituting open prisons for closed. We may no longer build high walls around institutions for the mentally handicapped, but we still surround them with bounded space, We build them in quasi-country, screened by trees, hedges, shrubs, gardens - the same screens we erect around our dwelling houses to sustain their privacy. New general hospitals also stand aloof. We do not see the use of cunning architectural tricks to blur boundary between public street and enclosed space as we might find in shop doorways, for example. Hospitals are a place apart. Again, it is essential to note that these new institutions may be a great improvement over those they replace. They may be far more comfortable environments. But they are no less insulating: it is merely that our architects have become more sophisticated.

In urban general hospitals in particular, we may find more emphasis on social boundaries as a way of erecting distance between hospital and its public. Outsiders may penetrate into the hospital on terms and conditions set by members of that organisation. For the most part, visiting is confined to restricted hours. Hospital schedules are out of phase with those most prevalent in the society. Furthermore, hospitals tend to be regarded as privy to certain mysteries, in the classical sense, which are not made visible to others. This, of course, is reinforced by the traditional reluctance of hospital staff to discuss their work with outsiders. Frequently they wear distinctive clothing and participate in a distinctive way of life.

We must be careful not to exaggerate this, however. There seems to be a certain trade-off between social and physical boundaries. As Clarke (1974) has shown, hospital staff *may* be deeply integrated into the local society; her illustration is drawn from a long-stay geriatric hospital housed in old Poor Law buildings, in an urban area, where nursing work in the hospital is seen to fall on a continuum with work in the local factories; but the same may well be true for workers in many of the large psychiatric and subnormality hospitals located in rural areas.

In general, then, I am suggesting that, as an instance of deviance, illness is normally managed by seclusion. So far as possible it is contained within the family as a private trouble. Where this option is not practicable it is contained within institutions organised to insulate the deviance from public concern and to limit the threat to public order. In this way the availability of alternative moral visions is restricted. Social control is of the essence of hospitalisation throughout the world. It is not the exclusive preserve of psychiatric hospitals in totalitarian states, although these may render such an aspect of hospitalisation more transparent.

Of course, we are also free to ask why illness as a form of deviance is handled by institutionalisation rather than redefinition. We do not, after all, find sickness rights campaigns which emphasise the moral desirability of sickness, as we do in the case of homosexuals, for example. This is basically a reflection of a moral consensus on sickness as a self-evidently undesirable state. Being sick is not as enjoyable for the sick person as sexual activity is for the gay person. Again, we must beware of ascribing essential qualities to the undesirability of sickness. This is a situational product. In particular, we must note that many of the experiences of the sick person may be much sought after in different situations. The disorientations of fever, for example, may closely resemble the disorientations generated by psychoactive drugs -

one can get as high on pneumonia as on cannabis. One might also suggest that we have a declining range of possible alternative definitions. Increasingly it seems that deviance can be subsumed only under crime or sickness and that other possibilities witchcraft, spiritual intervention, sin, bad taste, poor manners and the like are less and less frequently available. Redefinitions of deviance are restricted to the sickness-crime-wellness triangle. Non-Western cultures may be able to absorb some sickness by casting it as witchery with consequential effects on the patient. The attention of control agents may thereby be diverted from attempting to correct the patient's deviance by reclassifying it as non-theoretic and not open to patient-oriented intervention. If the condition is attributed to outside intervention, then there is no ground for holding the 'sick' person responsible. Attention must be directed towards other agents.

In this chapter I have attempted to set out a theoretical account of the relationship between illness and everyday life. I suggested that this could be done only against the background of the more general opposition between ordinariness and deviance. Both of these terms cover sets of sub-categories like health, morality and orthodoxy or sin, crime and illness. Ordinariness is seen as a moral condition that depends upon training, resources and effort. Successful presentation of oneself as an essentially ordinary person depends upon knowing what counts as ordinary conduct in oneself and others, upon the ability to meet these requirements and upon the motivation to make this commitment. Deviance is presented as a general term for breaches of the conventions upon which ordinariness depends, when no excusing conditions are available. The sanctions that are deployed vary with the degree to which the deviance is seen as motivated. Deliberate conduct is seen as deserving punishment; involuntary conduct, therapy. Particular acts may be categorised along this dimension, and of course bargaining may take place, as in pleas of mitigation or diminished responsibility. Illness is one category to which motivation is seldom imputed so that it presents a *prima facie* case for therapy rather than punishment. In some cases an ascription of illness may be sought to mitigate the due punishment for crime or sin, or the ascription may be withheld to incriminate the deviant as guilty. Examples of this are the borderline areas between kleptomania and shoplifting, nymphomania and promiscuity, battle fatigue and cowardice. All deviance is, by definition, a breach of some social order. No social order can be sustained without some system of deviance control by which members of the society can regulate each other's conduct within predictable limits. In the case of illness I suggested that families and hospitals were two of the key institutions for this purpose and examined the changing balance between them in terms of the changing relationship between public and private spheres of social life.

5   Illness and Sufferers

In chapter 4 I tended to concentrate on the social environment of the patient as the frame through which the possibility of sickness is made available to the sick person. I tried to set out something of the way in which social relationships, language and technology interact to generate the material and intellectual conditions for social action. But a constant theme of this book is that such matters cannot be separated from actual practical circumstances. Social order is a construct of dozens of individual instances of social action and cannot ultimately be divorced from them. Consequently, in this penultimate chapter I am turning back to the analysis of individual action to develop a tentative model for the study of illness as social action.

If we begin from some change in the relationship between the physical functioning of the body and the knowledge that we bring to bear to monitor that functioning, then I suggest that the use of Schutz's (1970; Schutz and Luckmann, 1974) discussions of relevance may help us to understand the issues involved. Ordinarily our physical functions and the knowledge used to monitor them are in some sort of balanced relationship that allows us to take our bodies for granted. They form part of the realm of the familiar, which is not consciously regarded or questioned in the routine business of everyday living. We do not commonly see walking, standing or breathing as everyday problems in the same way as we might try to decide whether a conversation overheard on a bus constituted teasing or abuse or whether a strange salesman was an honest man or a trickster. The familiar forms the predictable background against which the uncertainties of life can be identified, assessed and despatched. At times, however, even the familiar may become problematic or uncertain.

On the one hand, our knowledge may be refined, expanded or cast into doubt. In Schutz's terminology, there is a shift in our interpretational relevances. Those elements of our stock of knowledge, which we have previously regarded as applicable to interpret events, seem less reliable guides for action. There is, for example, a range of anecdotes about people reading medical books and becoming firmly convinced that they are suffering from every exotic condition described. Doctors and paramedical workers presumably experience a permanent modification of this relationship to enable them to cope with the balance between their own bodies and their expert knowledge.

More usually, however, the changes involved take place in the relatively autonomous biological systems involved in maintaining the normal functioning of the body. (At the risk of being repetitious, I would re-emphasise that these disturbances should be thought of as independent of the categories of Western medicine. For example, among South American Indians where dyschromic spirochetosis, which gives rise to various coloured spots of skin, was endemic, those who were 'healthy' by our standards were regarded as 'abnormal' and excluded from marriage.) Such changes may be due to deliberate human action, as in the ingestion of some pharmacologically active substance (not necessarily a so-called 'psychoactive' drug), or as a result of invasion by some hostile biological agent, as in infection, or due to some 'accident', like an apple falling on the head. These become imposed relevances, which arise 'from an enforced change of theme, which happens as a result of a break in automatic expectations (more generally: as a result of a cessation of life-worldly idealisations). The new theme intrudes in the form of something conspicuous and unfamiliar'. (Schutz and Luckmann, 1974, p.189). The more familiar and taken-for-granted these 'automatic expectations' are, for example the structure and functioning of the bodies we inhabit, the more salient and threatening disruptions seem to become. The classic account of this, in a rather different context, is Garfinkel's (1964) description of the consequences of his attempts deliberately to upset the conventions that maintain the stable character of everyday interaction and of the anxiety that this provoked in his subjects. This point is illustrated further in the empirical accounts reviewed later in this chapter.

The third element of Schutz's account of relevance relates to motivational relevance, which 'puts conduct in the current situation into a meaningful relation with life-plans and daily plans, in the case of both routine prior decisions and "extraordinary" decisions'. (Schutz and Luckmann, 1974, p.210). An actor's motives in a given situation lead him to select among the elements of that situation - a vast field of events is potentially available and competing for attention. He selects from these in the light of his current interests and projects. Obviously, this choice is not entirely free. Some elements may impose themselves by virtue of their unfamiliarity, as we saw above, or by virtue of the actions of others, which constrain the possibilities for one's own action. But there is always this element of competition between possibilities. In normal situations disruptions of body structure or function may readily become imposed relevances, possessing a high priority among the dimensions of a situation competing for the actor's attention. In extreme situations people may become unaware of these disruptions and they are pushed from their attention by the more urgent demands of other events. Many of the remarkable physical feats of explorers in hostile climes or of soldiers in battle or of disaster victims become more comprehensible when viewed in this light. The demands of survival impose themselves as more immediately relevant than the subjective experience of pain or discomfort. But such events are rare and, indeed, the depressed saliency of body events is one element that may be invoked to justify the identification of a situation as extreme.

This serves to underline the basic point about the priority accorded to disturbances affecting the body. These present immediate and important problems for the interpretive scheme being employed by the individual in any situation. The automatic expectation of a stable and predictable relationship between a person and his body cannot be sustained. If he is to continue to sustain a presentation of himself to others as an essentially normal person, who is sufficiently reliable to act as a competent partner in some encounter, then remedial action is called for. Such action is a three-stage process. Firstly, it involves an evaluation of the problematic experience in the light of the knowledge available to the subject. This allows him to identify what is going on and to note the courses of action made available by this identification - self-medication, visiting a folk healer, visiting an official healer, etc. It is important to emphasise however that identification does not necessarily entail recognising what is going on. It may be that the identification is one of ignorance: for example, although I do not know what is happening to me, this can still provide for action, as I consult those whom I think to be in a position to tell me. Secondly, the sufferer takes a decision to act. This may involve direct intervention by the sufferer as in self-medication or in direct appeals to local spirit agencies by sacrifice, prayer, fasting or whatever; alternatively, it may involve further consultation and a similar interpretive process on the part of advisers who may be official doctors, folk healers, priests or witches. This advice is then followed by some form of prescribed treatment. Thirdly, the effects of the treatment are monitored until the sufferer decides he has returned to a normal level of functioning. This is not necessarily the same point at which he started. It may involve a return to the physical *status quo* or it may involve amendments to the evaluative standards by which physical well-being is judged. A new balance may be struck between body structure and function and the knowledge used to monitor them. Alternatively, the sufferer may conclude that the treatment is not working and that a new evaluation is called for, followed by a possible new initiative in action.

The others with whom the sufferer interacts also play their part in these processes. I have already suggested (both here and in the previous chapter) that mutual monitoring of health status is an integral part of the general mutual monitoring of interactional competence in any social interaction. Where this is called into question, interaction partners may seek to impose changes in the relevance structure with which the other is operating. Such intervention may clearly have varying degrees of directness, from implications, through suggestions, to requirements. If someone's attention appears to wander while we are talking to him we may ask if he is feeling well and suggest that he sit down. If this is brushed aside and the other person subsequently passes out, we may feel obliged to require treatment by summoning medical assistance. The interests of others may also be taken into account in forming our own interests and our motivational relevance. Body disturbances may be selectively disregarded in situations that are not at all extreme where the interests of others conflict with our own interests in remedying this disruption. One account of a presumed myocardial infarction (Greene, 1971, pp.72-4), for example, tells how a doctor postponed attending to repeated attacks of severe chest pain from Christmas Eve until the day after Boxing Day in order not to disrupt the family Christmas. Cowie's data, discussed later, contain a number of similar examples.

A basic model for these processes is depicted in figure 5.1 . This proposes a general equilibrium between events in the biological sphere and events in the cognitive sphere. Such equilibrium need not be thought of as some single fixed point but as a range of normal variation. Our essential familiarity with our own bodies is not altered by the varying states of structure and function over the day between waking and sleeping. These regular changes in temperature, pulse rate, fluid balance and the like do not constitute disruptive elements in normal situations. The cognitive dimension contains both individual and social elements. By virtue of his unique biographical experiences, each individual participates in a particular fashion in the socially distributed stocks of knowledge available to competent members of the collectivities with which he is involved. Large elements of these stocks of knowledge must be held in common for social interaction to be possible; otherwise there would be no way of negotiating any working agreement, even on the meaning of the words used to negotiate that agreement. Nevertheless, each individual's version of that knowledge is in some way unique, by virtue of his unique experiences and plans, so that the application of socially shared

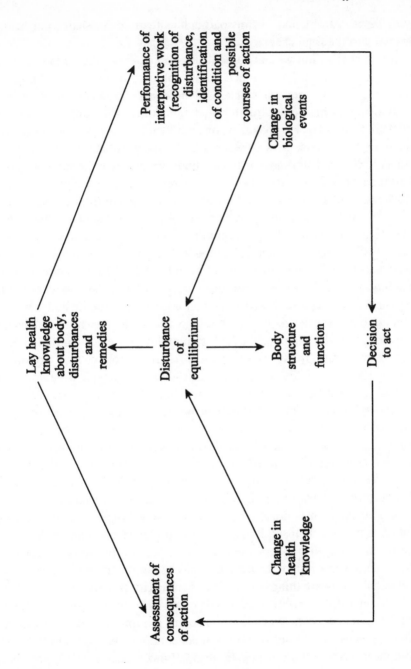

Figure 5.1 Basic structure of illness action model

knowledge is problematic in any particular situation. We shall come back to this point in the final chapter.

Into this situation we put some disruption of either the cognitive or the biological elements. I mentioned earlier the case of someone adding new knowledge to his present stock, which renders problematic his present relationship to his body structure and function. For example, reading an article in a newspaper or magazine on breast cancer may prompt questioning of the condition of one's own breasts. Alternatively probably more commonly some biological disturbance may take body structures and functions outside the range of normal variation. When there is a rise in temperature or an acceleration of the pulse rate the usual attitude of familiarity that we take towards our bodies must be suspended. As a consequence some kind of interpretive work must be performed to resolve these discrepancies. Such interpretation may be postponed temporarily if more pressing matters are to hand, but if the discrepancy persists I would suggest that it cannot be put off indefinitely. This is, however, an empirical question: we seek to reconcile the experienced changes with what is taken for granted about the body. We may explore our experience of the body to reconcile it with our changed knowledge. In the example above this might lead to self-examination of the breasts in a search for suspicious lumps. Alternatively, we may explore our knowledge of the body in an attempt to identify the typical nature of the biological disturbances we are experiencing. We may define them as a hangover, influenza, muscular strain or as something that we do not recognise and that requires further identification by someone with more specialised knowledge. Such interpretation is then followed by some action to restore a sense of familiarity whose effects are themselves monitored and evaluated. Unsuccessful action may lead into a repeat of the cycle. It is important to note that 'restoring a sense of familiarity' does not necessarily entail a return to the *status quo ante*. It may do, as when our consumption of magnesium carbonate remedies a stomach upset. It may however involve a recognition that things are never going to be the same again, as when we recognise cessation of menstruation as a sign of the menopause. The familiar monthly variations of a woman's body are things of the past. Familiarity is placed on a new basis.

Of course, this simplifies the actual processes in some degree. In particular the actual pathways between the decision to interpret and the evaluation of consequences are more complex than implied here. Some of these complications are brought out in figure 5.2. First, we can see the involvement of the others with whom the sufferer interacts. Invoking their own commonsense knowledge, including health knowledge, about individuals in

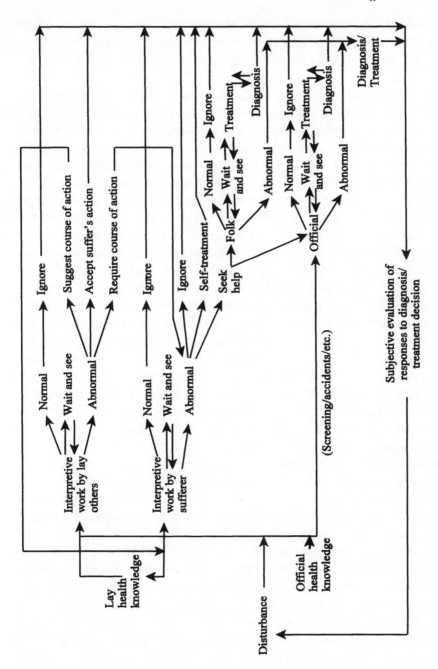

Figure 5.2 Some pathways through illness action model

their society, they are monitoring the membership competence of those with whom they are engaged in that encounter. If those others are perceived as normal, then they slide into the background of familiarity against which the encounter is set. (This definition of a condition of something as normal and to be ignored, like all the other similar decisions in figure 5.2, is provisional and open to revision in the light of new data.) Another possibility that recurs throughout the diagram is to wait and see. Judgement need not be made immediately. We may simply prefer to await further information. Finally, others may look for remedial action. They may, provisionally, accept the sufferer's own actions. Alternatively they may seek to impose action.

The force of this may vary with the status of the sufferer and the weight he attaches to membership competence in this instance. The relevance of some event for future action can be socially imposed only by coercion or by other members of some collectivity whose membership the sufferer values. I may suggest to a fellow passenger on a bus that he seeks attention for a bad cough. This carries little weight, however, since 'bus-passenger' is not a membership category that carries any great importance for most people. The implied charge of membership incompetence is not very critical for the business of living. The situation is different if I say the same to a colleague or a member of my family. Suggestion may slide over to requirement. There is, similarly, a dimension of coercion. Certain people in our society have recognised rights to coerce others. Parents and children form the most notable example here: parents have the right to define their children as ill and impose treatment regardless of the children's views on the subject.

We have already seen most of the relevant aspects of the sufferer's own decisions and interpretations. This model incorporates dismissal, self-treatment and help-seeking from folk and official sources. There is however a set of circumstances in which this may all be short-circuited. The principal events in this set are screening programmes and accidents. Screening programmes may reveal disturbances of which the sufferer is unaware, while accidents may create disturbances so suddenly that the sufferer is unable to act. Accidents may, moreover, short-circuit in two ways, either through the intervention of other laymen or through the immediate intervention of official medical agents. The latter applies particularly to accidents in public - car accidents, train or aircraft crashes, earthquakes and other natural catastrophes. In these cases we may find a relatively direct input of official health knowledge and official health services that we would not otherwise see until after a considerable amount of lay interpretation.

It is also worth noting that the 'wait and see' option becomes more complex in the case of both folk and official medical services when a distinctive diagnosis may not be established immediately but may be provided only after some treatment. A doctor may say, in effect, 'I don't know what you've got but if this medication clears it up, then we'll know it was probably that condition.' 'Wait and see' here does not imply quite the same thing as in the other contexts. Here it may include some definite therapeutic intervention, while elsewhere it implies only an openness to new information.

Since one of the avowed aims of this book is to stimulate research under the particular theoretical auspices I have been discussing and using the methodological approaches I shall be outlining in the final chapter, it is not surprising that there is a shortage of suitable illustrative material. Instead, I am required to rely more on the extension of arguments in other contexts, the re-analysis of other ethnographies and the disciplined use of my own commonsense knowledge about my own society. This allows me to illustrate and, I hope, illuminate particular features of this model, while denying me the opportunity for a fully comprehensive statement that might confer a stronger foundation to the model. My presentation draws particularly on literature that discusses psychoactive drugs, childbirth, polio and myocardial infarction.

Making Sense of it All: Psychoactive Drugs

The most extensive sociological discussion of the relationship between the operations of the human body and the knowledge on which attempts to make sense of them must draw is in the literature on certain psychoactive drugs. Although we are not dealing directly with phenomena that are commonsensically regarded as illnesses, we can still learn much about illness from them. Psychoactive drugs offer us a means of making a natural experiment on an individual's sense of the orderly character of his relationship to his own body and to the social world. As such they allow us to see, in a dramatic form, a paradigm for other extraneous disruptions of this relationship, resulting from the invasion of pathogens or the intake of some counter-invasive remedy.

The most comprehensive treatment of this argument is Becker's (1967) re-analysis of his earlier work on marihuana and its extension through a comparison with LSD. Becker notes the sharp controversy over the dangers of LSD use and the somewhat equivocal evidence of its effects. At this point the main debate on LSD was over its potential for precipitating psychoses. Becker observed that even if this potential were demonstrable it would be a unique instance of an identifiable single cause of a behavioural event. On the other hand, if we did not accept this view then we did have some responsibility to offer a better one that could account for these 'psychotic episodes'.

While the physiological effects of drugs can be ascertained by the direct intervention of the researcher in the relevant processes to examine, for example, the composition of blood, rates of heartbeat and respiration or changes in sensitive tissue - the subjective experience of the drug can be ascertained only by asking the subject how he feels. The two have no necessary relationship. The user may not interpret and respond to some of the physiological effects as drug-induced even if they are quite gross. Consequently, the same collection of effects may be experienced subjectively in a variety of different ways since each user may respond to different elements of the collection with differing emphases. In the particular case of recreational psychoactive drugs, their use is intended to give access to some subjective experience that is not available in the ordinary course of everyday life. Those effects that disrupt perception are most likely to be singled out for report. While these effects might seem uncomfortable or frightening to the outsider, they are none the less defined as desirable, pleasurable and worth seeking. The grounds for these interpretations are drawn in considerable part from the definitions of others whom the user believes to be knowledgeable. The interpretations that they make available provide a frame which the user can articulate with his own experience.

Becker comments on the rather vague status of the notion of a psychosis but elects to regard it as an alteration of relationships between the sufferer and his social environment such that the psychotic no longer shares the prevailing assumptions about his surroundings and is unable to engage in socially appropriate courses of action. This disruption is thought to be of a durable rather than a purely temporary nature. The perceptual changes induced by alcohol, on the other hand, are widely regarded as temporary and are not readily confused with psychotic symptoms. From this observation Becker goes on to argue that the reports of drug-induced psychoses generally come from inexperienced users. They take the drug and find that their perceptual world is disturbed, and do not necessarily attribute all the disturbing effects to the action of the drug. Such an experience shakes their confidence in their own normality. As Schutz (1962, 1964) pointed out, one of the basic ways in which we establish our own normality is by recognising that our perceptual world is, on the evidence available to us, isomorphic with the perceptual world of others. Where confidence in our grip on reality is shaken the categories that are made available to us by our participation in our own culture refer us to 'insanity' as a probable interpretation.

Where drugs are used in a context of interpretations furnished by experienced users, however, the consequences may be different. The novice user has available to him an alternative framework for making sense of his bizarre experiences and defining them as desirable or pleasant. As Becker (1963) showed in his earlier work, getting high was learnt - it did not follow automatically from the inhalation of marihuana. Other users can support the novice and explain what is happening so that he can be reassured of the temporary nature of his experiences and his essential normality. Non-users, such as physicians or journalists, who may be important sources of popular interpretations of these events, lack access to this specialised framework of interpretations and are likely to rely on the conventional ascription of 'insanity' to designate these events. The user who is not actively participating in a group of users subscribing to a special consensus may have only non-specialised interpretations available and can thus construct the experience only as a psychotic episode.

A natural history of the introduction of a psychoactive drug might involve a beginning phase when it is made widely available (along with information about usage) to users who do not have access to a pool of experience about its effects. No cultural frame is available to counter the ascription of 'insanity'. In this situation 'psychotic episodes' occur frequently. As a user culture develops, however, and knowledge becomes more widely disseminated, the number of psychotic episodes declines. Novice users learn the culture as they learn to use the drug. Becker argues that this model fits both marihuana and LSD. He notes that virtually all reports of marihuana psychosis date between 1920 and 1940 as marihuana became widely used in the United States. Although this statement is based on the published reports of physicians, and the decline may reflect only a change in reporting practice or publishers' judgements, it appears to bear out Becker's statement. Becker expects LSD psychosis to follow a similar course, although there are limiting factors: LSD is easily ingested and requires no special techniques like marihuana smoking or heroin injection. It may therefore be easier for a novice to obtain and use the drug without sharing the user culture. In fact the only interpretations available may be exaggerated popular accounts that might reinforce the frightening aspects of the experience. It is also possible for the drug to be administered to someone without his knowledge so that he cannot even ascribe the effects being experienced to the use of the drug. The novice may be able to anticipate the drug wearing off to provide an eventual release:

the ignorant have no such comfort and can probably decode the event only as insanity.

MacAndrew and Edgerton's (1970) work on alcohol reaches broadly similar conclusions. They note that conventional theories about the effect of alcohol propose a direct relationship between the physiological changes brought about by its action and changes in the drinker's behaviour. It is argued that alcohol removes inhibitions on conduct by depressing higher centres of the brain, which causes a loss of self-control. Such an argument asserts a causal connection between events in two separate domains - the domain of human physiology and the domain of everyday social action. The demonstration of such a relationship would require an exhaustive specification of events in each, a philosophically problematic task in itself and one that would not necessarily allow us to assert a causal link. The most one can say about disinhibition and drinking is that a hypothesis has been put forward that must be examined for its plausibility in the light of available evidence. Drawing extensively on ethnographic accounts, MacAndrew and Edgerton show that alcoholic beverages do not by any stretch of the imagination have ubiquitous disinhibitory effects.

This argument rests on two implicit and unexamined assumptions: it is assumed that all forms of alcoholic beverage and the physiology of all users are both perfectly substitutable. However, neither of these need seriously weaken the argument. Although alcohol does have a variety of complex interactions with other substances, it does not seem to be claimed that the nature of its effects varies drastically according to the form in which it is ingested, although absorption rates or the acuteness of the effects may vary. In the physiologists' view, it seems that alcohol is alcohol however it is disguised. Nor, so far as I am aware, is it seriously argued that there are radical differences in ordinary physiological processes between human populations. Individuals, of course, may have unusual metabolisms, but we are talking here in general terms, comparing one human group with another. As the authors note, there are definable and ubiquitous consequences in specific sensorimotor impairments, which allow us to feel confident that when we are discussing drinking in different cultures, we are talking about broadly similar beverages and reactions. But beyond this, a constant set of physiological events does not generate a constant set of behavioural events as the conventional hypothesis predicts.

One of MacAndrew and Edgerton's more interesting illustrations of their thesis is an extended analysis of the ways in which North American Indians learned certain styles of comportment when intoxicated. Conventionally,

Indians are regarded as notoriously unable to hold their liquor and the rapid decline of Indian social organisation and the demoralisation of individuals are commonly attributed to the effects of alcohol. Before the arrival and settlement of Europeans alcoholic beverages were unknown over large areas of North America. It has been supposed that on its introduction the Indians rapidly developed a craving for it and their behaviour became violently disinhibited. However, the earliest recorded accounts of the introduction of alcohol make it clear that this was not their initial reaction. On the contrary, the Indians remained largely peaceable and were often more frightened and alarmed than aroused by the unfamiliar experience. MacAndrew and Edgerton suggest that Indian responses to liquor were learned from their observations of European soldiers and trappers. These were integrated within Indian cultures, which already recognised fairly barbarous conduct towards each other and had socially legitimised time-out ceremonies, where the conventions of everyday conduct were suspended. The Europeans' drunken excesses were regarded as equivalent to these latter. The link between alcohol and socially legitimised disinhibition was a late development for the Indians.

Finally, one should also mention Castaneda's (1970, 1971, 1974, 1975) important work on his apprenticeship to a Southwest American Indian sorcerer. The early phases of this apprenticeship drew on experience with psychoactive drugs to furnish initial access to a separate order of reality. Castaneda learned how to use these drugs to alter his way of experiencing the world so that he saw it in terms of a special consensus about the reality and truth of these events. This consensus was shared among adepts. It was no more explicable in terms of some meta-language than is the ordinary consensus that sustains the everyday reality in which we mostly live. It could be experienced only in its own terms. Its logical structure was complete and self-consistent within its own set of justifications and its language made available analysis of that order of reality. This logic and language could not be translated into everyday logic and language, but merely described in a partial fashion. Castaneda's account shows how he fumbled towards this understanding as he attempted to make sense of his bizarre experiences in the terms that his master, Don Juan, made available to him. Finally, he became able to dispense with the drugs and gain immediate access to this separate ontological order, but this is beyond our present discussion. (I am aware that the factual status of Castaneda's account has been disputed. Personally, I see no good reason to treat it as fiction. I share Mary Douglas's (1973) view that it is an entirely plausible and deeply important piece of ethnography. However, even if it were fictional, its consistency with my general argument would still lead me to feel that this is the *sort* of account that we should be trying to write.)

How do these illustrations relate to our central interest in illness? Well, at the least, they suggest an important line of inquiry into the effects of pharmacologically active substances. Becker (1967), for example, notes that drugs ordinarily used in medical practice rather than for recreation, like adrenocortical steroids, are said to carry a risk of psychosis. He suggests that this may well also be the response to unfamiliar alterations in subjective experience which the user does not anticipate or connect with the drug and interprets as 'insanity'. This ascription may then be reinforced by the physician making a diagnosis of drug-induced psychosis, rather than interpreting the symptoms to the patient as common and transient side effects. But once we reach this point it is arguable how far the distinction between 'psychoactive' and other drugs is useful for sociological inquiry. If we accept the preceding argument that all drug-induced changes in the body are subject to cognitive interpretation, then they are all, in that sense, 'psychoactive'. Of course, we still have an interesting problem of determining under what conditions drugs can be classified as 'psychoactive' rather than falling into some other category. For instance, cannabis was widely used in Britain until recently for its effects on the respiratory system. Until the moral panic of the 1960s it would not generally have been regarded as a psychoactive drug beyond a rather esoteric circle of recreational users, medical researchers and those with experience in the East. The classification practices of physicians can, then, be seen as social phenomena deriving from the interpretive framework that they bring to bear on the physiological events their investigative techniques make available to them.

I have not, however, given this limited field such prominence merely in order to underline these two relatively trivial points, which are, in any event, somewhat peripheral to my argument. The importance of this work lies in its possible uses as a paradigm for the analysis of the social consequences of any physiological event. We can see the three types of relevance identified by Schutz at work here. The ingestion of some substance that disturbs the user's sense of familiarity with the structure and function of his own body may become an imposed relevance. The user can attempt to make sense of this experience by drawing on the stocks of knowledge that are available to him as a member of a number of collectivities. From among these he can select those elements that seem most appropriate to the sensations he is experiencing. Such elements may include what other users have told him or what he has read in newspapers and magazines or seen and heard on the

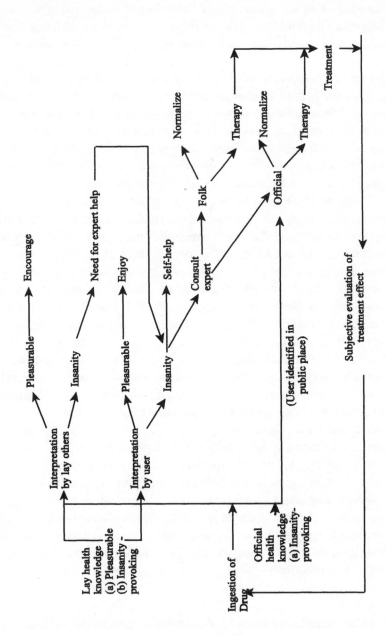

Figure 5.3 Recreational ('psychoactive') drugs

television or in the cinema. The assembly of these two elements - body changes and culture - hinges on the user's interests in the situation. Other features of the situation may have priority. This may account for the protestations of motorists that they are not drunk to a degree that impairs their driving. The demands of driving on his attention may simply leave the motorist unaware of the changes in his body structure and function. Similarly, where others are attempting to impose the relevance of changes and particular selections among interpretationally relevant knowledge, the degree to which this is accepted depends upon the degree to which the user values their association and wishes to continue to be recognised as competent in their eyes and, of course, on the degree of coercion that they can exert.

Some of these processes are represented in figure 5.3, which is a simplified version of the earlier model. In particular, I have omitted the 'Wait and see' options and the link between the equivalents of 'Ignore' decisions and the continuing review of the consequences of these decisions. Both of these continue to be relevant and the omission is merely for the sake of clarifying the remainder of the diagram. This shows how the ingestion of some drug is followed by an input of available knowledge to reach certain kinds of interpretations. In the case of recreational psychoactive drugs, shown here, the alterations in body structure and function may be taken as pleasurable or insanity-provoking. Where they are seen as pleasurable, the user can relax and enjoy them, unless and until unexpected or novel events occur. If they are seen as insanity-provoking then various remedial actions are available. These may involve self-treatment or the search for expert help from official medical agents or from locally recognised specialists, often experienced users. If the disturbance occurs in a public place, the condition may go directly to official medical agents and have an official definition imputed, in this case probably 'psychosis'. Both folk and official healers, however, may adopt a variety of tactics. They may intervene to give some counteracting drug to stabilise body structure and function or to modify the user's knowledge so that he can make sense out of his experiences and render them familiar and non-threatening. A new balance between body states and culture can be struck.

What Is Happening to Us? Polio and Myocardial Infarction

This section develops the previous arguments further through a re-examination of reported material on two specific illnesses: poliomyelitis in young children and myocardial infarction in middle-aged adults. I shall attempt to assess how far these reports are susceptible to this reconsideration and the degree to which they bear out the proposed model. In this sense, then, their credibility is perhaps less strong than if I had available data from a study conceived explicitly within this framework, but I hope they may have some degree of persuasiveness.

Davis's (1963) account of child polio victims is particularly important in throwing light on the social imposition of relevance. Davis pays relatively little attention to the children's perspectives on their condition, but the processes by which their next-of-relation sought to make sense of events can be seen as following the general pattern described above. This underlines the degree to which any ascription is an interpersonal construction. In discussing sickness as a subjective experience, we cannot neglect the degree to which validation of this experience and any consequent claims depend upon its evaluation by others. To a considerable extent, we recognise ourselves through the actions of others towards us, although this too is influenced by our own evaluation of others through an inspection of ourselves. 'Taking the role of the other' entails not merely seeing ourselves as others see us but also seeing others as we see ourselves, inspecting the typical knowledge, motives and interests available to us to determine the comprehensibility or rationality of their actions. The processes by which we evaluate others and they evaluate us are broadly parallel.

The data on which Davis's study is based were collected over a period of eighteen to twenty-four months after the admission of children with poliomyelitis to hospital and a diagnosis of moderate or severe paralysis. Fourteen families were involved. They were all white - and mainly working-class - residents of a single American city. Family members were interviewed and observed in encounters with medical and welfare services, and other ethnographic material was also collected on these facilities and their personnel.

Davis (1963, pp.15-29) describes the processes by which a diagnosis was reached. Initially, the children reported a feeling of physiological disturbance sore throats, stomach ache, fatigue, headache or some combination of these. This complaint was evaluated by the parents. In some cases, it was supported by parental observation of nausea, constipation, listlessness or a slight fever, and a common childhood ailment such as a cold, stomach upset or overtiredness was diagnosed. Alternatively, parents were able to account for the complaint by reference to some mishap, like a playground fight. Home remedies like aspirin or a laxative were prescribed and the child's activity restricted. Essentially, the parents initially regarded the child as suffering from some common minor illness that could easily be managed by home treatment. In three cases, however, where the parents could not validate the child's complaint by reference to externally available data, the child was accused of malingering to gain attention. This applied, for instance, to one child who complained of a stiff neck and had a history of such malingering.

However, as the illness developed, both of these sets of hypotheses became inadequate. The hypotheses could continue to be elaborated, although the charge of malingering was not sustained. Davis does not explain how this comes to be abandoned. Commonsense diagnosis provided for an interpretation of muscular weakness or rigidity in terms of a cold 'settling' in a particular part of the body or a 'weak spot'. Otherwise, the hypothesis was not doubted until the development of phenomena for which it could not readily account. Given the variation in the rapidity of onset of polio, this might arise within a few hours of the initial diagnosis or take some days. The key seems to have been a break in the child's normal relationship with the social world. Previously the child had been treated as essentially well, morally normal. The disturbance was a transient modification to this state. Now it was seen as a more radical alteration, since some markedly unusual event had occurred. In this instance we have what Davis calls symptomatological cues - failures of body management such as falling down, being unable to stand or dragging a leg - and behavioural cues - striking discrepancies in everyday behaviour. In the case of one child suspected of malingering, he was overcome by a younger sibling in a tussle.

Two other possible sources of doubt were recorded. First, parents were applying different kinds of knowledge to the initial observable physiological events. One family was quick to suspect polio because they knew that there had been several other cases in their neighbourhood. The possibility that their daughter's illness was serious was more immediately salient than in the case of most of the other families. Secondly, for some families the immediate remedial response to common illness was to call in the doctor. In these cases it might be the doctor who drew attention to the potential seriousness of an apparently straightforward condition.

Unfortunately it is not clear how the emergent incompatibility of the parents' theory about their child's illness with the events it purported to describe relates to the decision to seek help. One possible inference from Davis's account is to suggest that professional aid is sought largely as a consequence of this breakdown, but Davis himself is not clear on this point. However, we are left with a tentative account of the interplay between evidence of the state of body structures and functions and the knowledge available to the sufferer and those with whom he interacts. In these cases the child complained of feeling unwell, levelling a self-accusation of deviance. This complaint was inspected in the light of the available contemporary evidence and what was known about the child and his past. Where the self-accusation was validated, the child was attended to therapeutically. Although his behaviour might be conventional, theoreticity was not imputed and he was not held responsible. Where the self-accusation was not validated, the child might have both conventionality and theoreticity imputed and be accused of malingering. (This resembles McHugh's (1970) category of lying.) Theoretic deviance invites punishment. But these decisions are continually provisional. Any finality is merely for the here-and-now. As I suggested in the previous chapter, Davis found a bias towards normalisation. Parents attempted in the first instance to categorise this illness as a routine trouble, a ripple on a pool of essential health. In time the accommodations required to justify this became too great and the unusual character of the events was recognised.

We can see too something of the contextual character of events. Individual encounters are surrounded by permeable membranes that allow the past and the future, and the wider social context of the present, to penetrate. While these may all be expressed anew on every occasion their influence cannot be neglected. One of the great failings of microsociology has been its atomism. Societies may be constituted by myriads of individual encounters, but they are also constituents of those encounters. Something of this can be seen here in the way parents searched their child's past to account for his present condition whether in terms of an accident, a mishap, a disease contact or a known tendency to malinger. Similarly, some parents moved rapidly to a suspicion of polio in the light of their knowledge about events in their locality.

Cowie (1976) offers a more systematic treatment of some of these issues in his discussion of cardiac patients' responses to their condition. His sample were middle-aged men and women suffering from their first proven myocardial infarction. Sixteen out of the twenty-three patients initially applied a commonsense lay diagnostic category. The attributions depended upon the context in which the pain was experienced. Some identified it as a bout of indigestion, others as a recurrence of some illness, like gall bladder trouble, bronchitis or colic, and others put it down to an injury sustained at work. Only those patients who experienced sudden and severe pain immediately recognised this as a potential heart attack. The data available did not allow them to elect for a more favourable interpretation. One patient, for instance, said he knew it could not be indigestion because the pains were in the chest rather than the stomach.

> The symptoms ... were ... normalised in a variety of ways. They were regarded as indigestion which 'everyone knows' is a non-serious, non-threatening, common ailment treated by a variety of home remedies, or they were regarded as indicating the recurrence of yet another bout of a previously experienced illness which, although it may be serious, need not cause alarm as recipes for action had in the past proved successful. (Cowie, 1976, p.90)

The remainder of the sample immediately sought medical aid. Their pain had been sudden, acute and, most importantly, *unexpected*. They could not accommodate it within the causal context available to them.

The decision to call in a physician depended upon one of two similar phenomena: either an experience of physiological sensations that could not be accommodated within the interpretive framework available to the patient, or a break in the accommodation between interpretation and experience. This accommodation was based on changes in the quality and duration of the problematic experiences. The response of other family members was based on similar processes. 'Spouses claim to have realised something serious was wrong because their conception of their partner in his/her everyday normal activities or appearance was challenged ....' (Cowie, 1976, p.91). Their ongoing assumptions about the ordinary character of the social world and its citizens were disrupted by an inability to reconcile their observations of that world with the set of interpretations routinely available to them.

Cowie's account illuminates several features of the sufferer's self-diagnosis. Firstly, he shows something of the wait-and-see character of decision-making. Most of the patients initially applied some lay category amenable to self-treatment, if indeed they made a clear diagnosis. The decision to seek help is based upon a final recognition by the sufferer that the interpretive possibilities that he has at hand are exhausted. He cannot continue to recognise the physical sensations he is feeling as a familiar trouble for which remedies are readily available. Rather, his sensations represent an unfamiliar experience for which he lacks the knowledge to set up immediate remedial action. Secondly, Cowie also emphasises the way in which his subjects invoke the past, and their own ideas about the sort of people that they are, to form a context for the present events. Cowie (in a personal communication) suggests that people ask themselves two questions:

(i)   Can I account for this symptom by reference to my medical biography?

(ii) Am I the sort of person who could have/take X, Y, Z?

They may connect current health events back over months, even years, to a series of previous episodes that can be depicted as pointing towards this present condition. In identifying the condition sufferers invoke lay conceptions of 'at risk' categories, the types of people who could be afflicted by certain conditions. Cowie shows that others ask themselves similar questions about sufferers, as with the parents in Davis's account. Lay theories, as I showed in chapter 3, allow actors to analyse situations, disintegrate their elements and reassemble them in a wider causal context. Our sense of the continuity of the social world is founded on processes such as this, which bind individual encounters together.

The interpretive schemes invoked by both Cowie's and Davis's subjects, as competent members of Westernised societies, recognise sets of socially licensed problem-solvers, in this case doctors. These problem-solvers are people who have particular access to detailed specialist knowledge that allows them to engage in a wide variety of remedial actions in particular areas. From another stance, we can see them as agents for the maintenance of public order, since one aspect of their work is the containment of alternative versions of the social world, based on different interpretive organisations of material sensations. In yet another light, they act to set the world to rights for people who are troubled. Much of the debate about the politics of medicine, particularly psychiatry, misses this essential dualism. Psychiatry may be a moral and political enterprise. It is also about compassion to people in need of help.

If an individual's problem falls outside his knowledge and capacities for remedial action, then he is likely to turn to the problem-solvers licensed by the consensus among members of his society. Their view of the world is, like any other, partial, although it may often be presented in an absolutist form. This comprehensive system of explanation with its remedial prescriptions and failure conditions to justify lack of success may prove plausible to the troubled person, or be coercively enforced. Neither need occur, though, and the troubled person may set off a continuing search for help from other licensed and unlicensed problem-solvers. In our society, doctors are one kind of official problem-solver. Others might include police officers, clergymen, social workers and schoolteachers. Unlicensed problem-solvers might include faith-healers, clairvoyants, *mafiosi* or mediums. However, in a plural society, licensing may be awarded in a variety of ways by different groups who cannot be assumed to agree between themselves on the precise borderlines between the licensed and the unlicensed.

Scientific medicine offers a comprehensive system of explanations and justifications for failure, which doctors have particular rights to invoke. It tends towards exclusion of its competitors and annihilation, conceptual or actual, of alternative views. We can see this latter process at work historically in the suppression of American midwifery and the continuing hostility in both Britain and America towards 'fringe' practitioners like osteopaths and chiropractors. Scientific medicine has, as Freidson (1971) and others have noted, secured a fairly comprehensive monopoly over healing. This makes the search for help when licensed problem-solvers fail rather hard to document, although it is an area that might offer interesting possibilities for further research. It is easier to draw on anthropological material from contexts where there is more open competition between theories and practices of healing. It also allows me to underline the point that medicine is not necessarily *the* socially licensed problem-solver and that Western doctors may, in local terms, be the fringe, unlicensed, practitioners.

Press (1969) examined responses to illness in Bogota. He notes how most studies of Latin American medical practice have been based in rural areas where peasants have few real alternatives to folk medicine. In urban areas, however, 'folk' and 'official' healers may find themselves in direct competition as resources for the sick. Press describes how certain kinds of social and biological theories have different consequences in bringing the sufferer to the attention of official and unofficial healers, physicians or *curanderos*. Three elements are particularly identified. Firstly, in some cases physicians and *curanderos* are perceived as being in direct competition; either one may be selected as appropriate or both may be seen simultaneously. Secondly, in other cases compartmentalisation may occur where some conditions are defined as relevant to one system and others to the other. Thus, a 'folk' illness like 'susto' (Rubel, 1960, 1964) may be brought to a *curandero* while an 'official' illness like 'cancer' may be brought to a physician. Thirdly, patients may be influenced by considerations of the conduct appropriate for members of the social group with which they wish to claim or demonstrate association. Thus, those Bogotans who wished to show how 'modern' they were might invariably consult a Westernised physician, while those asserting traditional values might invariably consult a *curandero.*

Whatever the origins of their help-seeking decision, the sufferers' conceptions are renegotiated and refined in contact with the healer of choice as he assimilates them to the interpretive scheme that he has at his disposal. The outcome may be either 'successful' treatment as recognised by both parties or 'unsuccessful' treatment in the terms of either or both parties. The recognition of the success or failure of treatment is the outcome of a working agreement between patient and healer on what is to count as the outcome and what it will take to achieve it or, alternatively, on what are legitimate conditions for failing to achieve it. Such a consensus may evolve out of appeals to assumed-to-be-shared understandings, by explicit formulations of the knowledge owned by either party, with the aim of persuading the other of its acceptability, or by coercion. (This still involves some kind of consensus about what one party may invoke to threaten the other. Power grows out of the barrel of a gun through the shared understandings of aimer and target.) Where the biological events cannot be normalised, the sufferer may be freer to discard the interpretive scheme agreed with the healer, renounce the implicit or explicit failure conditions and seek an alternative.

Such a process is described by Schwartz (1969) as a hierarchy of resort. Among the Manus, from the Admiralty Islands, Melanesia, there was continuing competition between traditional and European medicine. While each system carried its own explanations for failure, which practitioners found complete and satisfactory accounts, these were not necessarily accepted by sufferers. The sick person might resort to a succession of healers within a number of theoretical systems in the hope of remedying his condition. The point of entry and the sequence depended on the sick person's interpretation of his condition and the causality that he imputed to it. Failure within one system of explanation and treatment might not be accepted but, rather, might lead to a review of the original help-seeking decision and a search for new sources of aid. The concept of a hierarchy of resort finds important echoes in the work of Sacks (1972) on the processes whereby suicidal persons came to contact a psychiatric clinic and Sudnow's (1967, pp.153-68) account of the chains of contact along which news of a family member's death would be passed. Both of these authors present us with images of social life in terms of interlocking membership of collectivities with consequent rights and obligations between members of those collectivities. Certain kinds of social events set in train searches among these relationships to identify who has the right to be told of a death first or the obligation to aid a potential suicide. Sacks presents the emergency psychiatric clinic as a last resort when all the relevant membership categories have been searched and found to be empty.

This emptiness is not merely a matter of there being no person available to fill the category, but of there being no *competent* person.

It should be possible to analyse the hierarchy of resort among socially licensed and unlicensed problem-solvers in similar terms. Licensed problem-solvers and those with problems are bound in particular relationships of rights and obligations. The failure of either party to meet these conditions without adequate justifications or excuses can exempt the other from their mutual obligations and turn their attention elsewhere. In *The Godfather,* for example, the father of an assaulted girl turns to Don Corleone for 'justice' when adequate retribution is not provided by the official law enforcement system. Similarly, patients may turn from scientific medicine if it is unable to deliver the promised remedies or produce justifications or excuses that they find convincing.

I have, then, tried to examine and develop the general applicability of the illness action model in the context of a number of empirical reports. I have attempted to sustain my argument that the observable patterns of conduct are the outcome of a continual process of interaction between the material world of sensation and observation and the ideational world of perception and interpretation. Illness action is the outcome of continuing efforts on the part of the sick person, and those with whom he associates, to make sense of what is going on in the light of the knowledge, resources and motivations available to them. We have seen how these interpretations draw on everyday knowledge of wellness and illness in attempting to resolve the divergence between body structure and function and the ideas that normally allow us to regard it as familiar and taken-for-granted. This everyday knowledge relates both to the specific instance of the disorder in question and to the individual's general picture of his place in the moral and social order. Both of Cowie's questions - on the nature of the condition and the nature of the sufferer - need to be resolved if familiarity is to be restored. These interpretive processes may span a period of time or be quite compressed. We may come to an immediate diagnosis or wait and see what develops. Our eventual diagnosis, too, has a provisional quality. It is open to refutation by new information or new events. Some diagnoses lead us towards various bodies of problem-solvers who are identified as relevant to the problem in hand. Some of these may be socially licensed, others not. They can be viewed as forming a hierarchy of resort as the individual searches the categories of action available to him for some competent remedy.

A Speculation: Childbirth

After the 'Is illness deviance?' debate, the 'Is pregnancy illness?' controversy must rank second among the hoary old chestnuts of medical sociology. Can a natural process that most women are likely to go through at some time in their lives satisfactorily be called an illness? Well, in my view, it all depends on what is meant by an illness. I noted earlier Fabrega's view that illness was necessarily a value term, since it was used to indicate a harmful deviation from some optimum. Pregnancy does not generally carry this negative evaluation, although pregnancy-in-a-context may. We can recall the old joke:

Doctor: I've got some good news for you, Mrs Brown .

Woman: It's Miss Brown, actually.

Doctor: I've got some bad news for you, Miss Brown. You're pregnant.

Even with a negative evaluation, however, pregnancy is generally categorised as social deviance rather than biological deviance. It is sin rather than sickness. On the other hand, there is no doubt that we are dealing with a condition that provokes radical changes in the physical sensations of a woman's body that are available for her interpretation. And pregnancy comes into the orbit of those control agents who are responsible for the management of relations between socially acceptable interpretive schemes and physical sensations. Pregnancy is regarded as the proper concern of the medical profession and its acolytes. In some ways an appropriate analogy may be more with the psychoactive drugs with which I began this chapter than with illness in a strict sense of the word.

The nature of the experience of childbirth is currently a topic of some controversy. The situation is particularly fluid in that both the physical sensations and the interpretive framework surrounding childbirth have been rendered problematic to an unusual degree. On the one hand, the physical sensations of childbirth are being radically affected by the activities of a number of prominent obstetricians exploring the potential of new technology for the active management of labour. It is argued that it is now possible to make the chance event of childbirth a predictable and well regulated process. Deliveries can be organised to occur at times when experienced staff are readily available, after a relatively short and generally painless labour. The progress of mother and baby can be continuously monitored and the obstetrician can intervene rapidly if either appear threatened. Intervention can help obstetricians to achieve their aim of a live, healthy baby and a fit mother as the outcome of every pregnancy by reducing both mortality and morbidity. It is also suggested that women find active management reassuring and that their anxieties about giving birth are reduced. They can be told fairly precisely when the labour will begin, how long it will last and when delivery will take place. They can feel that little has been left to chance and that there are few risks to either mother or child. The whole armoury of modern medicine is fighting on their side.

Against this, on the level of ideas, we have the arguments of a section of the Women's Movement that is concerned with the restoration to women of greater rights in their own bodies. They have been influenced by the theorists of Natural Childbirth and argue that many of the difficulties women experience in labour are a product of the threatening nature of hospital environments and birth technology. Women are made to feel anxious and threatened by a perfectly natural event and this, in turn, feeds back on the physical sensations of birth to amplify their painful and threatening nature.

The classic theorist of Natural Childbirth, in Britain at least, is Grantly Dick-Read. My prime source here is a 1958 copy of his *Childbirth Without Fear* which was originally published in 1942 and had gone through three editions and fifteen reprints and been translated into nine languages by that date. The prose is somewhat purple and unfashionably illiberal in many ways.

> Woman herself . . . is adapted primarily for the perfection of womanhood, which is, according to the law of Nature, reproduction. All that is most beautiful in her life is associated with the emotions leading up to this ultimate function. . . . From time to time, pestilence and war sweep through nations robbing them of much that is best in their stock. If we are to survive as a people, and as an Empire, we must constantly be alert, to improve our stock . . . Motherhood demands to be raised to its rightful position of pre-eminence in the affairs of State. (Dick-Read, 1958, pp.xi-xii)

But throughout Dick-Read has a burning humane concern with a central paradox.

> ... does Nature inveigle woman along the course of its essential purpose by bringing her first into contact with the irresistible demands of all that is beautiful? Is she led on and on from one joy to another by some force which intends to make her pay eventually the price of pain before she can achieve her

objective? If this is in keeping with the law of Nature, what can be its purpose? (Dick-Read, 1958, p.xi)

One of his biggest puzzles is that the more civilised a people are, the more intensified the pain of labour appears to be, although the fundamental anatomy and physiology of reproduction are the same throughout the human race.

He examines the efforts made over the centuries to relieve the pain of childbirth culminating in the widespread use of anaesthesia. Then he recounts the origin of his dissatisfaction with technological childbirth in the remark of a woman who had refused chloroform - 'It didn't hurt. It wasn't meant to, was it, doctor?' This led him to develop a theory of natural childbirth linking cultural images of pain and anxiety, transmitted from mothers to their daughters, by doctors and in the mass media, to overtense musculature in the tissues involved in childbirth which create a variety of obstetric difficulties. The remedies lie in deliberate relaxation and the conscious attempt of those involved with obstetric services to create a calm atmosphere.

The particular theory of muscular tension propounded here is unimportant to the present argument and I am not qualified to assess it. More interesting, however, are Dick-Read's other suggestions. Firstly, there is an implicit statement about the ease of parturition in non-civilised parts of the world. Put at its crudest, there is a prevalent notion that primitive women stop hoeing the fields, go behind a bush, drop the baby and go back to work and that it is all as simple as that. Nothing could be further from the truth. Thompson's (1967; Thompson and Baird, 1967b) work in the Gambia shows clearly that most births are obstetrically hazardous and that mortality and morbidity are kept within tolerable bounds only by the generally low birth weights of the babies. Labour was frequently prolonged and painful. However, there were strong cultural prohibitions against expressing pain.

> Keneba women are expected to bear their babies in silence, however long or painful a labour may be. Those who cry out are ridiculed and called 'cowards' and are reprimanded for prolonging labour and causing unnecessary inconvenience and trouble for everyone. (Thompson and Baird, 1967b, p.513)

Childbirth in Keneba was entirely women's work and men were excluded until some days after the process was completed. A number of women would be involved, especially the mother's female relatives and members of a group of old women who were thought to have special expertise. Births usually took place in the pregnant woman's hut or in her mother's, although a minority took place in the bush or in the huts of the 'specialists'. To the casual observer, then, we might have here a paradigm of natural childbirth and an exemplar, albeit without Western standards of hygiene, of the programme of women's health care groups: deliveries took place in familiar surroundings with the aid of fellow women and with a minimal intervention of men or of technology. The mothers' conduct displayed none of the anxiety or pain expressed by Western women. But Thompson is quite clear that even here labour is a most hazardous business and that suffering is not absent. It is merely closely controlled.

Apart from this fallacy concerning childbirth among the primitive, however, Dick-Read does make a number of interesting observations about the expectations women bring with them. He identifies five potential sources: respected others, those who have direct experience, the state of public opinion as expressed in the mass media, important historical accounts and the activities of experts. He notes that in the fifteen years between the first and third editions of this book the climate of opinion had changed little. Husbands, mothers, kinfolk and friends of the pregnant woman still present an image of labour as a painful and traumatic experience. Similarly, writers of fiction and newspapers tend to seize on the dramatic elements of births. Suffering makes good stories. Scientific writers furthermore separate the physiology of childbirth from its psychology.

> The whole act is described from the point of view of its mechanism; the impression we get is that the woman concerned, for the time being, becomes a machine, without either consciousness or volition ... We are never told whether the mother is likely to have any views, or whether the attendant obstetrician has any duties to perform at the upper end of the body as well as the lower. (Dick-Read, 1958, pp.57-8)

Attention is also drawn to the influences of the Judeo-Christian tradition and the biblical presentation of childbirth. Dick-Read demonstrates that there is an important error of emphasis in the Authorised Version of the Bible where the original translators have been led to insert references to pain in accord with the prevailing ideas of their times. This comes out quite well in the New English Bible with its better use of original sources. Compare these versions.

	Authorised	*New English*
Genesis 3:16	I will greatly multiply thy sorrow and thy conception; in sorrow thou shalt bring forth children.	I will increase your labour and your groaning, and in labour you shall bear children.
Isaiah 21:3	Therefore are my loins filled with pain; pangs have taken hold of me as the pangs of a woman that travaileth. I was bowed down at the hearing of it; I was dismayed at the seeing of it, and my heart panted; fearfulness affrighted me.	I am gripped by pangs like a woman in labour, I am distraught past hearing, dazed past seeing, my mind reels, sudden convulsions seize me.

Clearly, on these texts, pain cannot be credibly presented as a *necessary* concomitant of childbirth. The process may be hard work, confusing and bewildering, but it is certainly not violently painful. I do not take 'pangs', for example, as suggesting anything stronger than discomfort, and confusion and bewilderment are exactly what our model would predict, especially in an inexperienced mother who lacked a clear framework for making sense of her experience. Nevertheless, the teachings of the Churches have tended to follow these older interpretations, which undoubtedly reflected the contemporary situation, where childbirth was no doubt as painful and as hazardous as in Keneba, but where the pain could be directed into a spiritual context. The context of religious uplift through suffering provided for an emphasis on expressing the anguish rather than bottling it up as the African women did.

Finally, Dick-Read turns his attention to the activities of the medical profession. He points out that the need to seek medical aid is itself anxiety-provoking, since medical aid is associated with illness. People see doctors because they are sick. Having encountered medical services, the woman is then reduced to an appendage of her reproductive system. She is subjected to a battery of scientific investigation and then packed off home. Once labour begins, the woman is ushered into strange clinical surroundings, filled with masked figures and bizarre equipment. She is wired up and plugged in. Her body is arranged in a variety of unnatural and uncomfortable positions. Not infrequently, her participation in the process is limited or eliminated by anaesthesia so as to permit the obstetrician a free run. Obviously, this is something of a caricature, but like most caricatures it contains elements of truth. It is easy to see how modern obstetrics *can* be a very intimidating experience. But in some ways, there have been improvements. Natural childbirth theories have had some influence. Against this, however, is the technological revolution of recent years which makes possible, although not inevitable, assembly-line care. It is not the technology of active management of childbirth that should cause concern. It is the context of ideas within which it takes place. Used judiciously, the techniques of active management could significantly enhance the experience of childbirth, by further minimising the areas of risk.

I have discussed Dick-Read's ideas at some length not because of the intrinsic merit of his basic theory or indeed the evidence on which it is based. Most of it is entirely a matter of anecdotes and vague generalisations. This is not a problem confined exclusively to this work, of course: even recent accounts of pregnancy and childbirth, like that of Hubert (1974), do not go much beyond this. But it does have the merit of pulling together in one place the diverse factors that must be taken into account in any comprehensive analysis. In any study of responses to childbirth we need to examine the complex of ideas and experiences that turn around this singular event. Firstly, we must ask what the parties to a birth bring into the delivery room with them. In varying ways doctors, midwives and mothers all draw on lay cultures to make sense of events. These ideas are transmitted through the mass media of the society (television, radio, newspapers, books), through the official systems of ideological transmission (education and, to a lesser degree, religion) and through informal exchanges with kin and friends. The latter may draw both on their participation in the public net of ideas and on their own experiences. At this level, in particular, the system gains a degree of historical depth, since the experience of others is invariably in the past. Doctors and midwives participate, in addition, in a rather exclusive collectivity ordered by reference to esoteric and specialised knowledge that is generally unavailable to outsiders.

These provide the framework within which the experience of birth can be deciphered. That experience has, itself, three aspects. First, there is the observable conduct of mothers, doctors and midwives. Each is giving off a series of signals for the others to make sense of in the light of the knowledge available to them. It is easy, here, to see how a definition of childbirth as pain can be generated and sustained. Medical staff are likely to be in the habit of reading confusion, groaning, and so on as indicating pain in the person giving off these cues. This, presumably, will generate some degree of solicitude and the offering of analgesics or anaesthetics as appropriate responses. A woman who is receiving this type of attention may be cued into reading her own experience as one of pain since she is being treated as if 'pain' is the appropriate term to apply.

Parallelling this observable conduct, we have, secondly, the inward physical sensations being experienced by all the parties to the birth. In the case of the clinical participants these sensations are familiar and disregarded. For the woman giving birth, however, these sensations are *not* normal, although experienced mothers may come to regard them as routine. She can make sense of them only from the material she has at hand, her own advance knowledge derived from lay culture and, as above, the conduct towards her of others. Thirdly, we must also mention the physical nature of the setting. The maternity hospital presents a particular form of the organisation and identification of space. The nature of the rooms and their furnishings, decor, illumination or whatever set limits to the possibilities for action, although the determination of possible actions rests with the interpretive frameworks that participants draw upon.

All of these points are, of course, empirical questions, and my answers lie at the level of speculation. Nevertheless, I believe that the illness action model does provide the kind of theoretical underpinning that further inquiries require. It directs our attention towards the detailed study of the cognitive aspects of social action. We need to scrutinise the knowledge that is being involved in any encounter to make sense of the events in that encounter and to look at the ways in which this articulates with observable conduct. But I have said little so far about how we might actually carry out such investigations. I have criticised the theoretical and methodological bases of existing work in this area and argued for an alternative set of approaches. This theoretical programme is, however, decidedly vacuous if it does not attempt any prescription for research. In the last analysis its benefits or otherwise will be determined by the degree to which research under its auspices advances our understanding of the social world. It is to this that I turn in the final chapter.

6   The Way Forward?

In previous chapters I have tried to develop an account of the social aspects of illness. I began with a critical review of a selection of the more influential formulations of these issues and argued that the majority of these were, in various ways, both theoretically and methodologically unsound. In particular, I suggested that they displayed most of the characteristics of absolutist and scientistic thinking, in that the actions of research subjects were reduced to epiphenomena of social and psychological factors whose occurrence, relevance and import were legislated by the investigator. In contrast, I proposed that we should develop approaches that were articulated with the commonsense knowledge, or body of lay theories, which was invoked by actors to recognise what was happening, to formulate its relevance for their concerns and to act upon it. Illness was seen as a form of failure at everyday life, a disruption in the familiar and taken-for-granted balance between subjective experience of one's own body structure and function (or one's observation of the body structures and functions of others) and one's knowledge, as a competent member of some collectivity, of what is normal experience or conduct under the auspices of that collectivity. As a form of failure at everyday life, illness belongs to a set of events covered by the term 'deviance'. It has consequences for the maintenance of social order that are the concern of a variety of control agencies. These contentions have been illustrated through a reinterpretation of some available ethnographic accounts of disturbances of body structure and function.

It is, however, an easy game to pick holes in others' work; it is part and parcel of the everyday stuff of academic life. If this is to be more than an empty polemic, then its arguments must be turned into constructive suggestions that might point us towards productive research. This will be my principal concern in this final chapter. Disregarding events in the biological domain as the province of the life scientist, I intend to concentrate on tying the arguments in this work more closely to those in the general field of ethnoscience and to examine the methodological programmes that have been drafted for that field. I shall give an extended account of these prescriptions, although it will become clear that I do not fully agree with many of the claims

123

of its proponents. Ethnoscientists may be, and have been, as absolutist as anybody else. Our task here is to disentangle that which is of genuine merit and to see how this programme might be built on, rather than to accept it uncritically.

Ethnomedicine

Throughout this book I have taken the line that medicine, illness and the like should be seen, for sociological purposes, as folk activities. By attaching the prefix 'ethno' I have tried to keep this position in front of the reader. It is, of course, the case that we can take this stance in relation to both so-called 'folk' and so-called 'scientific' medicine. In sociological terms the theories used by both 'laymen' and 'experts' are accorded an equal status and their use is to be examined in parallel analyses. The medical knowledge invoked by the physician to interpret a patient's conduct is *formally* identical to the medical knowledge invoked by any layman to interpret any other's conduct. The study of ethnomedicine forms a special instance of the general enterprise of the study of ethnoscience.

As a term 'ethnoscience' describes both the knowledge that members of some collectivity draw on to find sense in their social and natural world and the study of the content and organisation of that knowledge. In this latter sense it is distinguished from ethnomethodology, which may be seen as the study of methods by which members of the society reconcile their theoretical understandings with their practical circumstances. Ethnomethodologists tend to ask 'How' questions. Ethnoscientists ask 'What' questions: '...ethnoscience tends to emphasise the static thingness of the phenomena being studied whereas ethnomethodology is concerned with the active process whereby things (mainly activities) are constituted in the world of social action'. (Psathas, 1968, p.514). Like most such distinctions this is a rather crude and artificial one. There has been a considerable degree of exchange between ethnoscience and ethnomethodology. Moerman's work, for example, features in anthologies compiled within both traditions (Tyler, 1969; Sudnow, 1972). However, it is a convenient distinction to make for my present purposes, although we shall return to the point towards the close of this chapter.

The study of the theories of body structure and function that members of a particular collectivity use to make sense of their own subjective experience and their observation of others may be called ethnomedicine. This may embrace ethnoanatomy, ethnophysiology, ethnopharmacology and so on. Of course, in one sense, it is still a culture-bound category. An East Coast Eskimo confronted with British practice in relation to bodily experiences might prefer to call it ethnoshamanism. However, we must take a terminology from somewhere and, provided we are aware of something of the ways in which it embodies a form of life, must make the best critical use of it that we can. We must keep in mind that our subject matter will embrace areas conventionally designated as 'magic', 'religion' or 'witchcraft', as well as the practice of 'scientific' and 'folk' 'medicine. At heart, though, we are dealing with a crucial practical problem for any member of any collectivity: 'What is happening to me and my fellowmen?'

One key requirement for our investigations, then, is a way of studying the content and organisation of the ethnomedical theories that members of a collectivity draw on to render actions and events into intelligible phenomena. We might adopt the traditional approach of the ethnographer and simply involve ourselves in the everyday activities going on under the auspices of that collectivity while recording what is said and done. Our written, tape- or video-recorded data are then systematically examined in an attempt to develop a rationale that can account for the observable conduct and towards which it can be argued that members must be orienting themselves if they are to generate this and only this conduct. The work of Frake, which I discuss below, is one example of such an investigation. However, there are certain difficulties with this approach in some contexts: it may be a very time-consuming exercise for some topics. And indeed ethnomedical theories may not be invoked very often except where one finds societies with some area of specialised practice by more or less full-time ethnomedical experts. In our own society, one might observe ethnomedical work frequently in hospitals or consulting rooms but rather rarely elsewhere. Obviously this structured distribution of invocations is not without interest, but it may present problems if we want to study ethnomedical work prior to contact with official health care agencies. It might prove very difficult to collect a usable body of data from observation in factories or schools or other organisations to see when ethnomedical theories are used.

The institutions of privacy that we looked at earlier may also create problems for ethnographers. In rural peasant villages in tropical regions most everyday activities may well take place in the open air. One can learn a great deal just sitting outside one's own tent or hut and watching. This is not a practical proposition in most industrial societies. Homes, factories, schools, hospitals and the like are all insulated to some degree from each other and from the scrutiny of outsiders. The ethnographer must find a warrant for getting in and then manage his presence very carefully. Families present particular difficulties in this respect, since the numbers of people involved are so small that unobtrusive observation is very difficult. They are, however, rather important for the study of illness as they appear, on the face of it, to be the locale for a great deal of the interpretive work surrounding this topic, since family members are so visible to each other.

As a consequence of these kinds of problems, ethnoscientists have given a good deal of attention to structured eliciting procedures intended to evoke systematic accounts of local knowledge. We shall look at these in more detail later in this chapter. Beyond this, we also need to examine the links between these theories as they are available to members of a collectivity and observable conduct. In their concern with the precise description of lay theories, ethnoscientists have neglected their articulation with social action. We are left rather in the dark about how the relevance of theories to events is decided and about the ways in which theories are used to provide for subsequent action. If we conceive of social conduct as the outcome of recognition, formulation and action, then the outer terms have been somewhat neglected in favour of the inner.

Ethnoscience

In contrast with traditional approaches in anthropology with their emphasis on the classification of societies, ethnoscience concerned itself with the study of classifications. The older approaches depicted monolithic unitary systems shared by the community of anthropologists into which societies were to be slotted, in terms of their modal personality types, their kinship system, their religious beliefs or whatever. The cognitive movement in anthropology discarded these interests in favour of an attempt to study how people organised and used their cultures.

> This is not so much a search for some generalised unit of behavioural analysis as it is an attempt to understand the *organising principles underlying* behaviour. ... Cultures ... are cognitive organisations of material phenomena ... [they] are neither institutions such as house type, family type, kinship type, economic type and personality type, nor are they necessarily, equated with some over-all integrative pattern of these phenomena. (Tyler, 1969, p.3, original emphasis)

The ethnoscientists interested themselves in two main questions: which material phenomena were significant for the people of some culture, and how did they organise those phenomena?

By this summary, ethnoscience would appear to fit our working category of pluralist approaches to social science. In practice, however, this commitment is somewhat diluted, in ways that resemble those of the interactionists discussed in chapter 2. Tyler (1969, p.4) notes that we may encounter systematic *intracultural* variations in the cognitive organisation of phenomena, as well as *intercultural* variation. For each class of phenomena alternative organisations may be invoked in different contexts. Cultural unity evolves from the relations between variant forms and their contexts, Variants are not deviations from some basic organisation. Taken together with the rules for their use, they form that organisation. Such a unitary description, which transcends the unique and individual models deployed by individuals, may however be available only to the ethnographer. Although members of the society may all perceive their culture as unitary, the particular conceptions of its content may be individually and socially distributed. The anthropologist may, however, be able to build a model that will generate these empirical variants. It is important to note that this does *not* presuppose a consensus model of social order. One of the strengths of this approach is its ability to accommodate social conflict in a way that harks back ultimately to Simmel's discussion of conflict as a social relationship.

Tyler's account is, in some degree, a rather selective construction of earlier thinking. Certainly, earlier writers on ethnoscience were less modest in their claims, and they significantly neglected intracultural variation. This was particularly true of some of the original workers on kinship, notably Lounsbury (1964a, 1964b) and Wallace and Atkins (1960). In part, this was a result of their reliance on secondary data, the limitations of which became more clearly recognised in later work, like Goodenough's (1965) paper on Yankee kinship terminology, where he explicitly restricts his account to a particular group of English speakers and calls for further systematic inquiry into the variations of terminology found in other communities. On the other hand, even workers with original data like Frake (1961) or Conklin (1955) tended to pass over the issue of disagreements between culture members, on illness and colour categories, respectively. There was a clear tendency to talk as if cultures were monolithic entities in the same way as some interactionists talked as if there were a monolithic symbolic order that governed everyday action. In taking this view as an *a priori* stance there was a danger of sliding into a form of absolutism in legislating a particular relationship between culture and social action while neglecting the contexts in which such work was being done. It could be made to appear as if the meaning of events was homogeneous for all competent members of that society, that interpretation was unproblematic and that the relevance of the frame being used was unbounded in time or space.

But this is not the case in the more recent work collected by Tyler (1969), notably the papers by Gumperz, Moerman and Tyler himself. These all lay considerable stress on the need to extend ethnoscientific inquiry to the contextual features of settings. Naturally occurring situations have dimensions in time and space that may be identified by participants as relevant to their intended courses of action. These features may structure the possibilifies for action or be structured by the individual's plans. An example might be the manipulation of pronoun usage where the *tu/vous* alternation is available to identify the degree of familiarity between the parties to an encounter. The parties' knowledge about encounters may provide for one usage rather than another, but this usage may itself be manipulated to presume upon a relationship or to snub another and to crystallise the nature of the encounter as something other than the parties had assumed. Wootton (1975, p.46) cites an example of the manipulation of the Russian *ty/vy* alternation at the close of Lermontov's novel, *A Hero of Our Time.*

> In the final scene, an aristocratic young lieutenant unexpectedly meets at an inn an older captain, a man with whom he had served on an isolated outpost in the Caucasus. The captain rushes forward, but the lieutenant speaks first: 'How delighted I am, dear Maxim Maximych! Well how are *vy?* 'But ... *ty ... vy?*' muttered the old man with tears in his eyes.

Recent work in ethnoscience clearly depends upon some notion of knowledge that is socially distributed, subject to contextual negotiation and variation and with an endemic possibility of conflict. However, as we saw in discussing the recognition of plural value systems by the interactionists, this does not guarantee that these do not retain a deterministic position in relation to social action. As long as we hold fast to this, we may risk reverting to an absolutist sociology. This is a point to which I want to return later in this chapter. For the present I am content to have established, at least to my own satisfaction, that ethnoscience does not entail absolutism, although it may have absolutist features. I want now to turn to an analysis of its methodological prescriptions.

Componential Analysis

Although componential analysis was originally developed in the context of kin terms, a rather esoteric branch of anthropology at the best of times, it was rapidly taken up as a tool for the general analysis of classificatory systems in many areas of social life. The principal source for literature on this topic is Tyler's (1969) collection, which, indeed, covers practically every key article on both componential analysis and ethnoscience up to that date. I rely here primarily on Frake's (1962) paper, which provided the original methodological statement for the programme.

Frake notes that one of the commonest tasks performed by ethnographers is that of getting names for things. This task is typically carried out by pointing to the constituent objects of some event, eliciting the native words for these objects and matching these to the ethnographer's own words. Frake gives an example: if an informant calls object X a *mbubu* and I call object X a *rock*, then *mbubu* means *rock*. But this does assume that 'things' are objectively identifiable apart from some cultural context. The task of name-getting is merely one of matching labels from different languages. This does, however, make the rather breathtaking assumption that all languages make the natural and social world available in exactly the same way, and that there is no difference in the ordering of the world, merely in the labels that are affixed.

It may well be more fruitful, then, to look for the 'things' that go with the 'words' rather than the words that go with the 'things'. In other words, we suspend our assumption of the absolute homogeneity of the world in favour of the investigation of the relationship between language and the order of natural and social events. Objects and events are seen as defined by some cultural system of concepts that is embedded in the language of the culture. Verbal language is seen as particularly important since significant events for members of a society must be readily communicable between them; otherwise co-ordinated action would become impossible, as would the transmission of the commonsense knowledge that defines membership within the society, and its subunits, to new members and the enforcement of the assumptions of everyday living on both new and existing members. We can also note that verbal language occupies a pinnacle in the hierarchy of communicative systems. All other systems body management, art and music are potentially translatable into verbal language and, indeed, must be so translated for any kind of theoretical discussion. Verbal language forms a meta-language for these other systems, while being simultaneously language and meta-language in relation to itself.

Verbal language is the pre-eminent human communicative system. It is flexible in its possible referents, productive in its ability to generate new ideas and novel ways of speaking, and efficient in that those features of life requiring most frequent communication tend to have standard and relatively short labels (Brown, 1965, pp.332-40; Brown and Lennenberg, 1954). Given, then, that communication about features of a collectivity and its environment tends to be linguistic and to be efficient, Frake proposes that the study of the referential use of standard responses offers a useful way of beginning the systematic description of cognitive systems.

Frake sets out an initial vocabulary for performing this analytic task. The basic building blocks are *terms* that designate *segregates*. 'Terms' are the standard linguistic responses mentioned in the previous paragraph. 'Segregates' are categories of objects. (For the sake of exposition, I am just talking about 'objects' here. It should be remembered that this does not necessarily imply a perceptual referent in the sense of a concrete, material thing. It may equally apply to an event, a relationship or an abstraction.) Not all categories, however, are segregates since they are not all distinguished by terms. Nor is it the case that terms match segregates on a one-to-one basis. Terms are chunks of speech that perform particular kinds of work and are not tied to particular linguistic forms. Thus, we cannot rely on simple linguistic analysis of morphemes, phonemes and the like to identify terms for us. In effect, our initial course of investigation depends upon an element of guesswork in which we attempt to identify terms from naturally occurring speech and then pursue the kind of rigorous elicitation described below.

When a term is applied to an object, that term is necessarily exclusive. It asserts that the object is A rather than B, C, D or whatever. But the set of possible alternatives is fairly specific in any naturally occurring situation. The term applied is not selected from a universe of all conceivable terms available to competent speakers of the language in question; it is chosen from a more or less finite set of alternatives. If we go back to our example in chapter 4, when we say that someone is 'ill', we are contrasting this with the term 'well', not with 'black', 'female', 'old', or other possible properties that we might impute to that person. Such a group of terminologically contrasted segregates forms a *contrast set*. The relationship of contrast is not the same as that of class exclusion. Categories may be mutually exclusive but can be said to contrast only when the difference between them is significant for defining their use. To take Frake's example, 'hamburger', 'hot dog' and 'rainbow' are mutually exclusive, but in attempting to develop ways of classifying hamburgers it may be necessary to say something about hot dogs while rainbows are quite irrelevant to this exercise in any naturally occurring situation that we can envisage.

Contrast forms a horizontal level of distinction between segregates. We can also identify a vertical dimension, which we might call *inclusion*. Some segregates embrace contrast sets at lower levels of generality, while forming part of such sets themselves at their own level. Thus, we can see that 'football' may form part of a contrast set with 'cricket', 'hockey', 'tennis' and the like at one level, while including a lower level of contrast between 'Association', 'Rugby' (itself divided into 'Union' and 'League'), 'American', 'Australian Rules', 'Gaelic', etc. Combining contrast and inclusion, we can produce *taxonomies*.

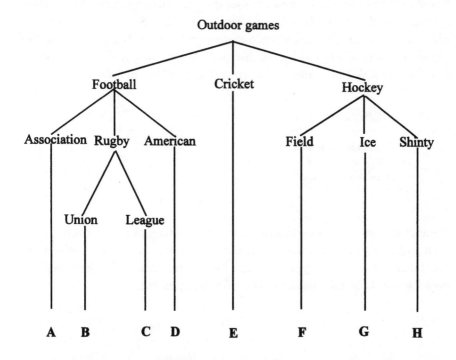

Figure 6.1 A taxonomy formed by partitioning the segregate 'outdoor games' by responses to events A-H

Taxonomies appear to be fairly fundamental to most human activity. They allow for the identification of objects and communication about them at several levels of generality in an economical fashion. They are a convenient way of ordering experience, and we can demonstrate that they appear to have some cognitive validity. For example, most languages provide some explicit method for moving up and down a taxonomy.

'Let's play a game of cards.' 'What kind of game?'

'Poker?' 'Five Card Stud, Anaconda, Fiery Cross?'

We shall return to this point of cognitive validity in a general review of these prescriptions. For the moment, we must also note that taxonomies do not carry any information about what it is that distinguishes one segregate from another or leads segregates to be subsumed under cover terms. The *components* of the segregate that are recognised in performing this task still remain to be identified. In order to do this, we must translate our taxonomy into a *paradigm*. If we take the example of the set covered by the term 'football' in figure 6.1, we can see that this includes the terms Association football, Rugby football and American football. For the sake of this illustration, let us suppose that these are discriminated by the shape of the ball round (R) or oval (O) and by whether forward passing is permitted (P) or forbidden (F). We can express the terms in the following formulae:

Rugby football	Fb, O, F
Association football	Fb, R, P
American football	Fb, O, P

Another way of expressing this relationship is in diagrammatic form, as with figure 6.2. This also indicates that boxes made available by the classificatory scheme may be left empty. In this case there is no kind of 'football' that has both a round ball and a prohibition on forward passing.

| | | Shape of ball | |
		Round	Oval
Passing forward	Permitted	Association	American
	Forbidden		Rugby

Figure 6.2 Paradigm of features for 'football'

Obviously this is a very simplified illustration, but it should make the relevant point. Having generated a list of the terms that apply to some specific area and their relationships of inclusion and exclusion, the analyst goes on to ask what features of the events are relevant to the decision to apply one term rather than another. What do we need to observe, for example, to be able to say that we are watching Association football rather than any other kind of football?

Two principal methods have been developed for generating data that may be susceptible to this kind of ordering. These involve either systematic elicitation procedures or the direct observation of naturally occurring situations. The former is generally accorded primacy as a source of data since it is easily reportable and replicable. One of the major problems of ethnographic observation has always been its non-replicable character. Here, it is argued, descriptions of the questions used to generate the data will allow any anthropologist to replicate the work.

Black and Metzger (1965) give an extended description of the technique of controlled elicitation in the context of field work on legal systems among Mexican peasants and American lawyers. They claim that their investigations are intended to reproduce the questions and answers that define conceptual systems and subsystems within particular cultures. This involves attempting to identify the things that make a difference in people's lives. To the extent that descriptive units are predicated on things that make a difference in some other cultural system, usually the ethnographer's own, this objective is defeated. However, one does have to start somewhere, in this case with Western legal categories, and discard this position as quickly as possible once an initial set of responses has been collected. The basic unit of inquiry is a question-and-response pair that is spontaneously produced by informants and remains stable between informants and over repeated eliciting from any one informant. These data are collected in a formal manner that is publicly reportable and replicable and turns essentially on monolingual eliciting in the language of the informant. By such means controlled variation of potentially significant stimuli can be introduced in an attempt to define the perceptual cues being used by members of the informants' culture to make inferences and plan action.

The elicitation procedure involves asking questions of informants. Black and Metzger emphasise that the significance of the responses can be assessed only in the light of the questions that they are answering, which may not be the questions the ethnographer posed. Human conduct, in general, can be seen as an array of responses to questions that people are asking and answering in every act. These are not easy to uncover because they are largely taken for granted: they are 'what everyone knows' without having to think. If the ethnographer is to describe the culture that his subjects invoke, rather than present a redescription in his own terms, he must learn the significant questions as well as observe the responses.

The ethnographer's approach is in some ways reminiscent of a child's. He starts to look for units that remain stable across a variety of contexts and appear to have a similar value. Two errors may arise here: similar forms may be identified as different, and different forms may be identified as similar. The ethnographer begins eliciting by developing some question in the native language and asking the informant to assess its grammatical and semantic status. The question can be tested by attempting to reproduce it across eliciting sessions and informants. As informants become more practised Black and Metzger suggest that they can be drawn into the production of questions: for example, 'What is an interesting question about ... ?' or 'What is a question to which the answer is ... ?' Or they can be asked to write a text in question-and-answer form on some topic of interest to the investigator.

The questions that are used in elicitation are made up of two parts. The skeleton of the question, the *frame,* is the most general form. Black and Metzger take an example from their study of American law:

'Does X take cases to court?'

The second part of the question is the *term* that is substituted for X in the frame. For example,

'Does the Attorney-General take cases to court?'

Where 'Attorney-General' is the term. In this instance the responses were not consistent and the frame needed refinement giving two further satisfactory frames:

'Does X press litigation?'

'Does X try cases?'

Elicitation is, then, self-correcting to some degree. Responses can, of course, also be used to construct new frames. Computerised retrieval systems can assist in organising and checking elicitation data so that gaps can be identified and inferences checked while field work is in progress.

By such means a corpus of data can be assembled that describes the usage of each term and maps it in contrast sets and inclusions with other terms. These data can be validated by using question-and-answer units to predict informants' responses. This procedure can be used equally for verification of correct pairs or falsification of deliberately incorrect pairs. The ethnographic description could also be employed to assess its correctness as an interpretive scheme, which would allow the user to be recognised as a competent member of the culture in question.

> ... it is obviously impossible to describe a culture properly simply by describing behaviour or social, economic, and ceremonial events and arrangements as observed material phenomena. What is required is to construct a theory of the conceptual models which they represent and of which they are artefacts. We test the adequacy of such a theory by our ability to interpret and predict what goes on in a community as measured by how its members, our informants, do so. A further test is our ability to behave ourselves in ways which lead to the kind of responses from the community's members which our theory would lead us to expect. Thus tested, the theory is a valid statement of what you have to know in order to operate as a member of the society and is, as such, a valid description of its culture. (Goodenough, 1964, p.36)

Two particularly interesting studies in ethnomedical areas using elicitation techniques are those by Metzger and Williams (1963) and Stark (1969). Metzger and Williams studied the activities of 'curers', lay healers, in the Chiapas region of Mexico. Having identified the general attributes of the class of people called 'curers', they developed eliciting frames that allowed them to generate the local classification of types of healers, the tasks each performed and the circumstances in which their help might be sought. They argue that the discriminations used are consistent with those used by indigenous speakers in natural situations. The scope of Metzger and William's interests makes a concise exposition of their methods and the relation to the data generated rather difficult, so I shall concentrate here on Stark's work, which, although more limited in its aims, allows us to see the principles of elicitation in practice.

Stark was interested in the naming of body parts by Quechua speakers. She mapped their terms for body parts into a taxonomic structure of part-whole relationships, ordered by what she termed relations of partiality. This is essentially the converse of the more common usage 'inclusion', which I described earlier. Her method began by the ethnographer pointing to some part of the body and asking the informant to name it. This could elicit several responses that were clearly not homonyms with identical points of reference. If the informant was given the frame, in his own language,

A is part of B

a variety of combinations could be identified which would allow for the mapping of relationships where some terms included others and their arrangement in a hierarchy where specificity increased as we descended. Each term belongs to one and only one level and is in complete contrast to other terms on the same level. The scheme terminates when informants disagree on naming and are evidently using a description rather than an established term. As Stark notes, this whole enterprise can be carried out with little or no appeal to semantic criteria. Terms can be mapped without direct knowledge of their exact referents. The precise detail of Stark's findings need not concern us here, but it is notable that the method allows us to assemble a description of Quechuan accounts of the body without reference to our own culture's descriptions. The area of reference is, however, still left rather hazy. This is particularly so since Stark is not really interested in moving from a taxonomy of body parts to a paradigm that might set out the distinctive features employed by her informants in naming.

By far the most relevant work for an examination of ethnomedicine, however, is set within the other tradition I identified, that of the study of naturally occurring situations. The study in question is Frake's (1961) work on disease diagnosis among the Subanun, a Philippine people. Frake concentrates on diagnosis as his focus of interest to avoid the complications of aetiology and therapy, which draw on both herbal remedies and supernatural influences, passing through religious specialists.

In most places, Frake observes, illness evokes such questions as: 'Am I sick?', 'What is wrong with me?', 'What can I do about it?' and 'Why did it happen to me?' Every culture furnishes a set of such questions, which may be asked by its members of themselves and each other in response to apparent bodily disturbances, of potential answers and of procedures for linking questions and answers. The cultural answers to questions about what is happening are *concepts* of disease. The information that is needed to eliminate alternative possibilities and establish a definite answer is the meaning of a disease concept. Sickness is a frequent topic of conversation among the Subanun. Hence, disease concepts are verbally labelled and readily communicable. Medical knowledge is not esoteric learning but is widely shared among the whole community, adults and children. Frake's study begins from actual identifications of 'being sick' and the questions that the Subanun themselves ask. The replies are examined to see what might be relevant for discriminating one member of a contrast set from another. Among the questions asked are, inevitably, a set that requires a 'disease name' as its answer (establishing a diagnosis). Such diagnosis is a necessary prelude to the selection of 'therapy' and the formulation of a prognosis, to a patient's future courses of action in general.

Diagnostic categories (disease names) are conceptual entities with a problematic relationship to any given instance of illness. These categories classify symptoms, stages of illness and what is to count as recovery. The course of any particular illness may not correspond to that of any diagnostic category and may require successive or simultaneous application of a number of disease names. Frake demonstrates that specific diseases are grouped together to form categories of kinds of disease that are assembled into taxonomic hierarchies. Again, the ethnographic details are relatively unimportant for my present purposes.

What is particularly important, however, is Frake's analysis of the linkage between disease names and actual cases of illness through the use of criterial attributes. Merely listing the members of a category does not tell us how they are recognised as similar or how they are distinguished from other categories. The cognitive saliency of the ethnographer's formulations remains to be demonstrated. Frake argues that there are three approaches to this issue that allow for the specification of analytic, perceptual or explicit rules for identifying names with objects. Analytic rules of use are ethnographer's rules. They depend upon an independent, etic coding system, such as phonetic or kinship notation, to code instances of an event and derive necessary and sufficient conditions for category membership. (See also Wallace and Atkins, 1960, pp.75-9.) But this is very different from furnishing a cognitively valid account, although it may enable the ethnographer to fulfil Goodenough's criteria for good accounts, quoted above. Secondly, one can attend to the perceptual cues that informants appear to use when categorising. Establishing these with any certainty seems a formidable and probably insoluble problem since there is no way in which we can get inside the heads of our informants, although it might be possible to make some progress in limited areas like colour categories (Conklin, 1955).

The only alternative is to ask informants about meanings: 'What is measles? How do you know it is measles and not chicken-pox?' This furnishes the ethnographer with the culture's definitions of the segregates concerned. Such definitions furnish explicit verbal criteria for identifying the attributes of members of some category that are particularly relevant for distinguishing that category from others. It was this method that Frake adopted for the analysis of Subanun illnesses. There was no reliable etic coding system. Western medicine is itself a culturally situated theoretical system and its use would confuse the basic issue of developing an account of

Subanun theories and the features to which they themselves appealed in making their diagnosis. There is no reason why disease classifications should be isomorphic. The limitations for ethnoscientific inquiry of treating Western medicine as a privileged theory are well illustrated by Lewis's (1975) work in New Guinea. Paradoxically, Lewis seems to have been handicapped rather than aided by his own training as a Western doctor, which seems to have made it very difficult for him to take native theories seriously and his account therefore shuffles uneasily between views of these theories as defective Western knowledge and as systems to be examined in their own terms.

If etic coding was not available to Frake, neither were perceptual cues. This reflects three particular difficulties stemming from the nature of the topic under investigation: first, since diseases tend to be scattered in time and space in their incidence, it is difficult to bring examples together for contrast and comparison (as might be possible for kinds of plants or animals); secondly, many diseases such as 'headache' and 'migraine' referred to internal states that could be distinguished only by verbal reports and where diagnosis was also affected by the social setting in which the report was made; thirdly, as non-material entities, diseases are not available for ostensive definition; that is to say, you cannot just point and say, 'That is measles' in the way you can say, 'That is a table'. Of course, the Subanun themselves faced similar problems, so they have to rely on verbal descriptions of significant attributes and have no difficulty in agreeing on disease definitions, although the articulation of these definitions with any particular case of illness remains problematic.

Frake's attempt to elicit diagnostic criteria paralleled those that he used to collect disease names. He asked informants to describe differences between diseases and to explain why particular instances were assigned to one category rather than another. He observed Subanun 'case conferences', at which diagnostic discussion took place, and noted the corrections that were made of his own diagnostic efforts. Like other classifications of natural phenomena, Subanun disease categories were conceptually exhaustive and widely shared. All cases of illness were potentially classifiable. A Subanun might say that he did not know the particular disease name but never that there was no name. Given the widespread interest in illness, disease information was available throughout the society. It was public knowledge on which there was general consensus at the theoretical level, although not necessarily at the practical level of actual cases of illness. Diagnosis played a central part in the cognitive organisation of illness, providing for the selection of relevant herbal remedies and for the prognostic and aetiological decisions that determined the form of 'religious' intercession that would be necessary to restore health.

The claims of ethnoscience are summed up by Frake (1962, p.86). He notes that they should provide the investigator with 'public nonintuitive procedures for ordering his presentation of observed and elicited events according to the principles of classification of the people he is studying' The accounts that can be given are both replicable and subject to test by falsification. By such means a rigorous description of cultures can be achieved. 'Culture' here is used in the sense given by Goodenough:

> ... a society's culture consists of whatever it is one has to know or believe in order to operate in a manner acceptable to its members, and do so in any role that they accept for any one of themselves ... culture is not a material phenomenon; it does not consist of things, people, behaviour, or emotions. It is rather an organisation of these things. It is the forms of things that people have in mind, their models for perceiving, relating and otherwise interpreting them. As such, the things people say and do, their social arrangements and events are products or by-products of their culture as they apply it to the task of perceiving and dealing with their circumstances. (Goodenough, 1964, p.36)

Methodological primacy, in this context, is accorded to the kinds of formal elicitation described by Black and Metzger (1965). Frake (1961, p.206) is almost apologetic for his reliance on traditional ethnographic observation, and his (1962) summary presentation of ethnoscience stresses the importance of formal methods, although he does emphasise that these cannot satisfactorily be completely divorced from direct observations. He takes a harder line on importing initial response-eliciting devices than do Black and Metzger, arguing that it is illegitimate to use any frame that is not used by the informants themselves. Instead, frames should be developed out of observations and then applied.

It is important to note two things about this approach, which its key exponents have not always brought out as clearly as they might. First, it is not necessarily an absolutist approach. It has on occasion been implied that the structures discovered by the ethnoscientist are unitary and homogeneous for all members of the culture in question. Although variant answers have been reported to eliciting questions, the tendency has always been to discount these. The practical aim of the investigator has been to produce a model that offers a single 'best fit' for the observable data. I would contend that this is an illegitimate assumption of something that should be taken as an empirical problem. There is no reason why this type of inquiry should not be used to investigate the structured social distribution of folk knowledge. Can we discover systematic differences within any particular society that might constitute discriminable collectivities bound together by the invocation of distinctive theories? Of course we can, if our basic samples are large enough. One of the principal weaknesses of ethnoscientific elicitation has been its reliance on very small numbers of informants, which would also tend to minimise intracultural variation.

Secondly, ethnoscience is a description of invocable knowledge on particular occasions. Again, this point is not always made clearly. There is a danger of translating monolithic or pluralistic accounts of invocable knowledge into the language of central value systems or external symbolic orders. This knowledge does not *determine* social action; it is used to *generate* it. The distinction is important. On this model it is not necessary to view human beings as epiphenomena of system activities. This point will be elaborated further in the following section when we review the ethnomethodological critique of this work.

I have outlined this approach at some length. In part, this is a conscious attempt to remedy the neglect that this important body of thought has received on this side of the Atlantic. However, an account at this length is also necessary if I am to set out an intelligible critique of this line of inquiry. Although, as I have indicated, I believe it has certain merits, I believe that its bases have not been adequately explored and that there are serious questions to be raised about the status of its reports, particularly over the issue of the linkage between the general descriptions presented and the specific instances of phenomena that they purport to describe. This is a central question for any theory and method and one that must be resolved if we are to succeed in our aim in explaining illness as social action, but it is an undeniable Pooh trap for unwary Heffalumps. Accordingly, the next section is devoted to a detailed examination of this point in the light of recent sociological writing.

Some Problems with Ethnoscience

For present purposes the criticisms I am most interested in are those set out by two anthropologists with a heavier debt to ethnomethodology. Lawrence Wieder and Michael Moerman. The approach has been vigorously debated in more conventional terms in the pages of the major American anthropology journals. Berreman (1966), for example, argues that ethnoscience dehumanises those it purports to study and is subscribed to basically by people who do not like other people very much. He prefers accounts that give a greater role to empathy. It is, however, precisely the repudiation of empathy in favour of systematic inquiry that lies at the heart of sociology as a disciplined study of social life. Unrestrained empathy is the province of the novelist or the propagandist. What distinguishes sociology from fiction is the constraints of standards of evidence within which the sociologist must operate. Ethnoscience does not supersede empathy; it disciplines it. Harris (1974) attacks ethnoscience as excessively idealist. This account, however, falls victim to the common traits of vulgar Marxism in assuming that material factors can directly affect social action and that phenomena such as power can be divorced from the circumstances in which they are identified. Technology, natural environment and coercion, as I have argued earlier, all depend upon interpretive work for their practical significance. The material world does not determine the world of ideas.

Wieder (1974) identifies two main groups of ethnoscientists. On the one hand, there are those like Floyd Lounsbury and, to a lesser degree, Ward Goodenough who have tended to work almost exclusively on kinship. On the other, we have people like Harold Conklin, Duane Metzger and, particularly, Charles Frake, whose work I have described at some length. Both groups have in common the position that language embodies a world view (the well established Sapir-Whorf hypothesis) and that semantic aspects of language are like grammatical aspects in that they are governed by rules, where 'rule' is used in the sense of a programming rule or a game rule. This latter feature is drawn from transformational linguistics, which attempts to specify a set of deep rules that will allow for the generation of grammatically correct sentences. Rules, in this sense, are conceived of as an exhaustive set of instructions that specify in advance what is to be counted as correct conduct. The proposals of the ethnoscientists presume that it would be possible to determine the meaning of an object or event for a member of a given society by analysing the semantic rules of the language used by members of that society. Wieder, however, notes that if we construct a model of the sort of society that this analysis presumes, the consequences are patently absurd.

The theoretical positions of the two groups of ethnoscientists differ sufficiently for us to need rather distinct models to exemplify their approaches. For the present discussion it is not very important to go into detail about the work of the first group, but it is useful to give a brief account of their model. Wieder identifies this as a *theory of corresponding marks,* in which there is a one-to-one relationship between language terms and perceptual objects. As marks, language terms exhaustively describe the perceptual world, which ceases to exist as any kind of independent phenomenon. On this reading, language *is* social reality.

Such a position, Wieder argues, has a number of rather odd consequences:

(i)   members of the society in question are no more than courses of talk. A silent member would have no existence and the society as a whole would consist of the sum total of the talking that was going on;

(ii)   the only distinguishing features of any object (or event) are those that society members talk about as evidence that the name of the object has been correctly applied. Since these features constitute the object, they define its interests for the individual, who cannot, then, initiate interests of his own;

(iii)   when a name is used, its only referent is the set of rules for its correct application. There is no reference to any visually perceived world;

(iv)   socialisation would consist of learning the names of objects and their distinguishing features by being taught those names with those features. Where a name had not been learnt, the object could have no significance;

(v)   speakers would be differentiated only by pronouncing their name, or having a name attributed to them, or by the character of their utterances, or of the utterances directed towards them;

(vi)   occasions would be differentiated only by naming them or by the character of the utterances pronounced within them;

(vii)   correct usage of a name would be defined only by consistency between the name/object and the features by which it is distinguished. Since the perceptual world is not available as a reference, no lies, in the sense of deliberate false naming, would he possible;

(viii)   again following from the lack of an autonomous perceptual world, there are no perspectives on events. All actors employ the same semantic rules and identify objects and events in exactly the same fashion. Intersubjectivity - ascertaining the relationship between my view of the world and yours - is not a problem.

As Wieder concludes, such a model describes no known society. He argues that it might apply to non-perceptual entities, such as gods, ghosts or demons but I think even this is doubtful since such entities are normally conceived of along parallel lines to human beings. In consulting an oracle, for example, if there is no reply, I suspect the inference is drawn that the spirit is silent or absent rather than that it does not exist. Some quasi-corporeal existence is implied apart from the talk. A more familiar example might be a radio play, which is a society composed entirely of talk. Yet even here the listener is required to perform a good deal of filling in to make sense of what is going on. He has, for example, frequently to hear some characters as present in the situation being presented although they are not actually speaking at that point. Again this trades on the listener's ability to assume a corporeal perceptual world tokened by the talking that is going on. In the context of our present discussion, this model would imply that illnesses existed only as names. Biological events and processes would be irrelevant except in so far as they were named as distinguishing features for attributing illness. There would be no problem about making identifications since all parties would be following the same semantic rules and forming the same perspective on events.

Some of these absurdities are removed by the other group of ethnoscientists in applying a *theory of corresponding tokens,* which restores the autonomy of the perceptual world by treating language terms as a limited set of names available to society members and applicable to an unlimited set of objects. In this position the rules for the correct application of names become less important. Correct usage is defined by reference to the fit between the name and the perceptual object rather than to the rules for correct application. As long as the name and referent coincide, there is little need to show the methods by which the name was applied. These do not function as the referent, as they do in the other version. Nevertheless, it does remain true that the relevance of an object for courses of action is determined by the distinguishing criteria that could be pointed to if the application of the token were challenged. The observer of an act of naming has to assume that these criteria were correctly applied, although he cannot know this specifically. Variations of method are inconsequential, provided that both actors' and observers' interpretive schemes require the same 'inputs' and produce the same 'outputs'. Each must make use of similarly available information and produce similar answers. This however allows that several different componential analyses of the same data may prove equally valid: we cannot produce a unique description of the way in which the name comes to be applied. Burling (1964) shows how the number of possible ways of dividing even a relatively small number of terms rapidly becomes astronomical. It is not at all clear how the appropriate arrangement is to be selected and how others are ruled out. We can also note that the restoration of autonomy to the perceptual world means that lying becomes possible, since there are external events against which token application can be matched.

This is the general model that Frake (1961) seems to be using in his work on Subanun disease and its diagnosis. As he records, 'The "real" world of disease presents a continuum of symptomatic variation which does not always fit neatly into conceptual pigeonholes.' The Subanun have a set of disease names that is considered as both finite and exhaustive (except when faced by 'foreign' influences) which they apply to a rather vague and indeterminate field of events. At the same time, however, Frake's ethnographic fidelity brings out the difficulties of his model.

To appreciate this we need to realise that a theory of tokens renders invisible the schemes of interpretation, the criteria for the application of tokens. These methods must be discovered anew by each society member. There is no theory of socialisation, which is accounted for merely in terms of experimentation, playing around until acceptable responses are produced. But this does not seem to fit any known society. It is quite clear that examples can be given to novices to exemplify criterial principles that make the employment and use of rules explicit and publicly available. As Frake notes, Subanun children learn about diagnosis through verbal descriptions of how to match disease names with distinguishing criteria. So it seems that rule usage is not as invisible as it is made out to be. At the same time, it is clear that the programming-rule model of the theory of marks is inadequate, although it does make rule usage more explicit.

This compels us to face a more basic problem with ethnoscience and componential analysis. The approach involves using names as a set of ideals that are matched against the world as it is perceived and experienced. It would appear from this that names mean exactly the same thing on every occasion that they are used and are employed in entirely standard ways in the light of standard prescriptions. What we are faced with is that quest for the Philosopher's Stone of fixed and determinate meaning criticised so cogently by Wittgenstein (1972) and his followers. In practice, as ethnographers have repeatedly found, names do not have a stable meaning but are matched against phenomena by an elaboration of the sense of the name or its distinguishing criteria to absorb each particular instance. Bloor (1976), for instance, in his examination of adenotonsillectomy decision-making, argues that the general criteria to which consultants subscribe take on specific manifestations for each individual consultant to which they refer in making a decision on any particular case. Although ENT surgeons might share a common set of names to use in their work, each of them gave a relatively specific interpretation to that set of names, which could itself be elaborated to match names and cases as necessary. Drawing on the writings of Bishop Berkeley, Bloor is relying on a somewhat different philosophical base from that of this book, but his conclusions are similar:

> Berkeley argued that the conceptions men frame, while they may be communicated as de-contextualised abstractions, are nevertheless not framed as abstract ideas but rather are always particularised and specific. The various routines of each specialist can therefore be seen as referring to a series of *specific* ideas of those signs, symptoms and circumstances for which surgery is indicated, with each specialist differing from his colleagues as to the nature of these specific ideas. Given these inter-specialist differences in their specific ideas of appropriate indications for surgery, then it is possible for specialists to differ markedly in patient assessments even though they might reach a wide measure of apparent agreement on appropriate indications where these indications are debated and communicated in abstract terms. (Bloor, 1976, p.45)

Frake himself reports similar findings for the Subanun. While there was a high degree of consistency in verbal definitions of diseases, these did not extend to their application in any specific case. Informants might agree that two different types of ulcer differed by their depth of penetration, for example, but disagree on which type was exemplified by any particular instance with which they were presented.

Any identity between one use of a name and another is not a logical identity. It is something that has been achieved, for the practical purposes of the moment, by a series of *ad hoc* elaborations. The criteria for using a name - the rules of correct usage - are similarly indefinite, although they achieve a working degree of determinacy in any particular situation. This is an important and much neglected point. While the meanings of terms may not be available in the homogeneous fashion assumed by componential analysis and may require some degree of filling in on each and every occasion of use, this indeterminacy is more of a problem for analysts of the social life of a collectivity than for the members of that collectivity who are actually engaged in the business of everyday living. In our everyday life the world is in order as it is and experienced as massively real, stable and predictable. We shall come back to this issue in the concluding section.

Before that, however, I would like to indicate one possible route out of this impasse of indefiniteness. This can be found in the work of Moerman, particularly his (1974) analysis of ethnicity as an interactional accomplishment. He inverts the issue of mapping criteria for the use of names by arguing that names are selected first and criteria are then adduced to justify this selection. The meaning of the name is the justification(s) for its use. Ethnic labelling is not some kind of conditioned response to certain traits, but a selection of a particular identification that is called for by the nature of the setting. This identification can then be defended by elaborating a set of criteria that might justify its usage. In Moerman's work, the Lue of Thailand point to a variety of cultural traits as distinguishing them from other neighbouring tribes. To the outsider, many of these may appear to be common to all parties, but the Lue can still appeal to them by identifying them as, for example, copies by others of a Lue trait. I have attempted a similar analysis of the term 'profession' as used by health visitors (Dingwall, 1976). Some of Frake's (1961) data are also amenable to this kind of construction. He quotes the case of an inflammation of his leg. Frake himself identified this as an 'inflamed wound' which he thought originated as a minor cut. The Subanun diagnosis however was 'inflamed insect bite'. When he contested this, it was argued that he had simply failed to notice the original bite. 'In such cases, the existence of the prodrome is deduced from its criteriality to a diagnosis originally arrived at on other grounds.' The Subanun were producing a justification for their decision. Moerman notes that justifications form lists, which have the property of being open-ended. Hence, an exhaustive specification of the use of a name is not possible. Nevertheless, in practice, the number of justifications that occur regularly may be fairly small and predictable. One possibility, then, might to be to regard the 'criteria' identified by componential analysis as justifications, which are drawn in a specified context from those that are regularly available. While it may be difficult to bring eliciting contexts into a known relationship with natural situations, this is not impossible and is a feasible empirical task. Elicitation may well give us usable approximations that can be refined in field observation.

Conclusions

In this version, then, the findings of componential analysis are seen as idealisations of what society members are actually doing. The sophistication of the analysis governs the relevance of the findings to any particular context. Clearly, elicitation is a much cruder device than observation. It takes us much further from naturally occurring settings and the links between culture and social action. On the other hand, there are some things that are difficult to observe. They may take place rather rarely, in private or in dyadic situations, all of which present particular problems for fieldworkers. Elicitation can paint broad outlines relatively quickly, although its findings are likely to be limited in their application to any particular setting. The significance of this depends very much on our interests. Personally, I am unhappy about the idea that the only things we are likely to be able to generalise about are structural properties of settings, divorcing the accomplishment of the forms of social order from the content of the particular order in question. Clearly these two issues are only analytically separable, since, as the preceding account has suggested, each can be used to criticise the other's tendencies. The ethnographer cannot afford to neglect the arguments and findings of the ethnomethodologists and vice versa. But there are many worthwhile tasks to be accomplished besides the kind of conversational analysis that some British writers have been attempting to legislate as the sole concern of ethnomethodology. The structures that generate intelligible conversations perform many other kinds of work. As Harvey Sacks saw, for instance, (unpublished lecture notes, 6 February 1970) turn-taking is not just about two parties taking turns to speak; it can also be mobilised to demonstrate the pattern of rights and obligations between them. Some principle specifying who goes first (or last) is available as a status marker, expressing one party's dominance over the other. Conversational structures do much more than generate orderly talk. There is an important second strand to ethnomethodology, which operates at a slightly different level to ask what is achieved by the methods that produce orderly conversations. This programme, articulated particularly by Churchill (1971) in analysing Blau and Duncan's study of the American occupational structure, calls for nothing less than a comprehensive ethnography of everyday life. Churchill argues, for example, that if we want to know how occupational structures, social mobility and the like actually influence the course of social life, then we should look at the occasions when they are actually invoked as relevant dimensions of natural situations rather than relying on expounding our own commonsense theories in legislating social reality for individuals.

However, such occasions (for instance, when ethnomedical theories are invoked) are likely to be relatively uncommon, and it may be difficult to witness a comprehensive collection of them. In such cases, elicitation techniques can be very useful short-cuts to quick and crude first approximations of the content and organisation of actors' knowledge. There has been no serious attempt in Britain to reproduce and extend any of the work in this area. Replications of the work of Frake and Metzger and Williams could tell us a great deal about the distribution of ethnomedical theories, about conceptions of problems and their socially licensed solvers and about the factors that are involved in generating observable conduct. Provided that we are clear about the status of what we are getting, there is no reason why this enterprise could not readily be undertaken. Obviously there are imperfections, as with any research method. But the generally acknowledged deficiencies of survey research, for example, have not stopped it from conferring important practical benefits on our public policies. Here, we are offered a significant advance in sophistication with an instrument that might allow us to plot and describe ethnomedical theories in a rigorous fashion without making the kinds of imputations that survey research entails. Such an account could have important consequences for health education programmes, which, it seems to be generally agreed, work best when they are clearly articulated with the intended recipients' present state of knowledge and present concerns. This kind of investigation can provide accounts of this knowledge, which are undoubtedly sufficiently reliable for mass education programmes. It can produce something that is true for most people most of the time, which is all health educators need to know for their purposes.

But there are, as we have seen, clear limitations to what one can do with such formal methods. Apart from anything else the eliciting process may still impart a sharper structure to the data than might otherwise be the case. We need to see theories at work and to be able to examine precisely how they are linked with observable social action. I remain to be convinced that it is an illegitimate enterprise to observe naturally occurring social action and to present some sort of account of the implicit theories that parties appear to be drawing on to make sense of the event. There have undoubtedly been difficulties with this in the past and I think that new standards are required.

Previous ethnographers have been too ready to substitute their readings of events for more direct and faithful reproductions. They have described conversations, for example, rather than reported them and allowed us to judge for ourselves the appropriateness of the inferences being made.

Admittedly, there has been something of a fashion for theoretical nihilism lately, which argues that one can, in principle, make almost any kind of inference one likes and that no one inference is better than any other. This debate, on decontextualised meanings, presents an endless source of fascination for armchair fieldworkers. it is, however, based on a clear fallacy and a misinterpretation of linguistic philosophy. If one has ever done any serious field work, one thing is patently obvious: meanings are not problematic for competent actors. Indeed, this is precisely how we recognise their competence and how we recognise the adequacy of our own field work. When situations become as transparent to us as to the other people involved in them, then we can claim to have understood what is going on. Taken in context, it becomes quite clear what inferences are permissible and one comes to share, with the individuals under study, the information that is available to justify one's inferences. This includes working background knowledge, the social and historical context of the observed encounter and a barrage of paralinguistic material. When one divorces descriptions or talk from this context, as is inevitable in any report, obviously these fragments can offer much amusement to the facile critic. And, in truth, there is no way to demonstrate conclusively that what the reporter says is how it was. All that can be done, really, is for the reporter to attempt to establish his good faith; to give grounds why the reader should believe what he says to have some ring of truth.

On the other hand, if we can be brought to trust the ethnographer, there is no reason why we cannot accept his reports as a definite account. Our critic may claim that he can think of twenty-seven different interpretations for any conversational extract we quote in our report. The fact is that that extract had a definite meaning for competent parties to the situation reported. Admittedly, that meaning may have required a lot of work to establish, but for that situation it was quite determinate. Problems can arise when we move away from particular situations in search of generalisation. Here, we must concede an element of indeterminacy about the social world. But if we keep hold of this point about the practical determinacy of meanings, then we can sharply minimise this problem. Provided that our reports respect the definite meanings that were actually applied, there is no reason why these cannot be collected together to make more or less general statements. We can quite properly say: 'This group of people see events like this and are likely to do this under these boundary conditions, which they see in this light.' The more exhaustively we can fill in these terms, the less practical indeterminacy we find. As Bloor (1976) argues, in his account of the relevance of Bishop Berkeley's thought to ENT decision-making, the more closely we can specify abstract ideas, the less problematic their application to any particular instance becomes. The 'Know-Nothing' party have missed this essential tension in linguistic philosophy. While Wittgenstein may argue that social meanings are potentially infinite, he readily concedes that they are practically finite, that the world is 'in order as it is'.

Ethnographic accounts might also add a useful corrective to the cognitive bias of most of this approach to social life. One of the principal achievements of contemporary sociology has been the restoration of rationality to areas of social life that have been stripped of intelligibility by the absolutist moralities enforced by public control agents. Throughout the present account I have insisted on the rationality, within the appropriate context, of apparently bizarre conduct. But this rationality can be misinterpreted as elevating the cognitive above the affective elements of social life. This may not be an unfair picture of the lives of the sociologists who have formulated these approaches. As intellectuals, we naturally tend to intellectualise problems. Other people's lives, and our own for that matter, tend to become objects of a rather cool and critical detachment. Our partisanship is moved by intellectual rather than personal sympathies. We should not, however, be blinded by this to the genuine distress of those whom we are seeking to study. Pain, suffering and death carry powerful emotional charges. Cognitive sociology may help us to explain them. It should not involve us in explaining them away. The apparent objectivity of social events may appear epiphenomenal to us; to others it is massively real and massively painful.

Such practical problems require practical remedies. If such efforts are not to go off at half-cock, however, they must be founded on an adequate theoretical understanding. The problem with so much research on social aspects of health and illness is that its humane concerns have led to a neglect of theory in favour of hasty empiricism. This problem is not unique to this area of inquiry. Many investigators of practical social problems have been similarly moved and the net result has been a hotch-potch of pseudo-science that has signally failed to deliver the goods. My hope in writing this book has been that it may contribute towards shifting the grounds of future inquiries. *Social* problems and *sociological* problems are not the same thing, but if we are to make any constructive contribution towards solving the latter, we must first get our ideas straight on the former. Theorising should not be left to become some arid and self-indulgent pastime of armchair sociologists. It is a necessary preliminary to any worthwhile practical empirical inquiry or social programme. It is every bit as relevant to the researcher or the policy-maker as it is to the speculator.

I would not be so bold as to claim that this book offers a conclusive or comprehensive programme. I am acutely aware of the unanswered questions and the unpursued hares it has put up. As E.A. Ross said many years ago,

> I am not wedded to my hypotheses nor enamoured of my conclusions, and the next comer, who in the true scientific spirit, faces the problems I have faced, and gives better answers than I have been able to give, will please me no less than he pleases himself. (Ross, 1901, p.ix)

I cannot improve on that as a statement of a scientist's creed. What I am firmly convinced about, however, is that no useful purpose will be served by further inquiries into the social aspects of health and illness without a clear conception of what it is that is being studied. And, if we are to achieve such a clarification, then the debate must shift to the levels to which this book has been addressed and to a programme of research that is founded upon self-conscious theoretical reflection.

Bibliography

Apple, D. (1960) 'How laymen define illness' *Journal of Health and Human Behavior* 1: 219-25.

Ariès, P. (1973) *Centuries of Childhood*, Harmondsworth, Penguin.

Barnes, J. A. (1969) 'Networks and political process' in J. C. Mitchell (ed.) *Social Networks in Urban Situations*, Manchester, Manchester University Press.

Baumann, B. (1961) 'Diversities in conceptions of health and physical fitness' *Journal of Health and Human Behavior* 2: 39-46.

Becker, H. S. (1963) *Outsiders*, New York, Free Press.

Becker, H. S. (1967) 'History, culture and subjective experience: an exploration of the social bases of drug-induced experiences' *Journal of Health and Social Behavior* 8:163-76.

Berelson, B. (1952) *Content Analysis in Communications Research*, Glencoe, Ill., Free Press.

Berger, P. L. and Kellner, H. (1964) 'Marriage and the construction of reality: an exercise in the microsociology of knowledge' *Diogenes* 46: 1-23.

Berreman, G. D. (1966) 'Anemic and Emetic Analyses in Social Anthropology' *American Anthropologist* 68: 346-54.

Birdwhistell, R. L. (1973) *Kinesics and Context*, Harmondsworth, Penguin.

Black, M.and Metzger, D. (1965) 'Ethnographic description and the study of law' *American Anthropologist* 67: 141-65 (reprinted in Tyler, 1969).

Bloor, M. J. (1970) 'Current explanatory models of pre-patient behaviour - a critique with some suggestions on further model development' M. Litt. thesis, University of Aberdeen.

Bloor, M. J. (1976) 'Bishop Berkeley and the adeno-tonsillectomy enigma' *Sociology* 10: 43-61.

Blum, A. F. (1970) 'The sociology of mental illness' in J. D. Douglas (ed.) *Deviance and Respectability*, New York, Basic Books.

Blum, A. F. and McHugh, P. (1971) 'The social ascription of motives' *American Sociological Review* 36: 98-109.

Brown, R. (1965) *Social Psychology*, New York, Collier-Macmillan.

Brown, R. and Lennenberg, E.H. (1954) 'A study in language and cognition' *Journal of Abnormal and Social Psychology* 49: 454-62.

Burling, R. (1964) 'Cognition and componential analysis: God's truth or hocus-pocus?' *American Anthropologist* 66: 20-8 (reprinted in Tyler, 1969).

Castaneda, C. (1970) *The Teachings of Don Juan*, Harmondsworth. Penguin.

Castaneda, C. (1971) *A Separate Reality*, Harmondsworth, Penguin.

Castaneda, C. (1974) *Tales of Power*, New York, Touchstone.

Castaneda, C. (1975) *Journey to Ixtlan*, Harmondsworth. Penguin.

Churchill, L. (1971) 'Ethnomethodology and measurement' *Social Forces* 50:182-91.

Cicourel, A. V. (1964) *Method and Measurement in Sociology*, New York, Free Press.

Cicourel, A. V. (1973) *Cognitive Sociology*, Harmondsworth, Penguin.

Cicourel, A. V. *et al.* (1974) *Language Use and School Performance*, New York, Academic Press.

Clarke, M. (1974) 'Getting through the work' Presented to BSA Medical Sociology Group Conference, York [Published in R. Dingwall and J. McIntosh (eds.) *Readings in the Sociology of Nursing*, Edinburgh, Churchill Livingstone, 1978.]

Conklin, H. C. (1955) 'Hanunoo color categories' *Southwestern Journal of Anthropology* 11: 339-44 (reprinted in Hymes, 1964).

Coulter, J. (1974) *Approaches to Insanity*, London, Martin Robertson.

Cowie, B. (1976) 'The cardiac patient's perception of his heart attack' *Social Science and Medicine* 10: 87-96.

Davis, F. (1963) *Passage Through Crisis*, Indianapolis, Bobbs-Merrill.

Dexter, L. A. (1962) 'On the politics and sociology of stupidity in our society' *Social Problems* 9: 221-8.

Dexter, L. A. (1964) *The Tyranny of Schooling*, New York, Basic Books.

Dick-Read, G. (1958) *Childbirth Without Fear* (3rd edn.), London, Heinemann.

Dingwall, R. (1974) 'The social organisation of health visitor training' Unpublished PhD thesis, University of Aberdeen.

Dingwall, R. (1976) 'Accomplishing Profession' *Sociological Review* 24: 331-49.

Dingwall, R. (1977) *The Social Organisation of Health Visitor Training*, London, Croom Helm.

Douglas, J. D. (ed.) (1970) *Deviance and Respectability*, New York, Basic Books.

Douglas, J. D. (1971) *American Social Order: Social Rules in a Pluralistic Society*, New York, Free Press.

Douglas, M. (1973) 'Torn between two realities' *Times Higher Education Supplement* 15 June.

Dubos, R. (1959) *The Mirage of Health*, New York, Anchor Books.

Dubos, R. (1965) *Man Adapting*, New Haven, Yale University Press.

Edgerton, R. B. (1968) *The Cloak of Competence: Stigma in the Lives* of *the Mentally Retarded*, Berkeley, University of California Press.

Elliott, H. C. (1974) 'Similarities and differences between science and common sense' in R. Turner (ed.) *Ethnomethodology*, Harmondsworth, Penguin.

Engel, G. (1960) 'A unified concept of health and disease' *Perspectives in Biology and Medicine* 3: 459-85.

Erasmus, C. J. (1952) 'Changing folk beliefs and the relativity of empirical knowledge' *Southwestern Journal of Anthropology* 8: 411-28.

Fabrega, Jr, H. (1972) 'The study of disease in relation to culture' *Behavioral Science* 17: 183-20.

Fabrega, Jr, H. (1974) *Disease and Social Behavior* Cambridge, Mass., MIT Press.

Fabrega, Jr, H. and Manning, P. K. (1972) 'Health maintenance among Peruvian peasants' *Human Organization* 31: 243-56.

Fagerhaugh, S.Y. (1973) 'Getting around with emphysema' *American Journal of Nursing* 73: 94-9.

Foucault, M. (1973) *The Birth of the Clinic*, London, Tavistock.

Frake, C. O. (1961) 'The diagnosis of disease among the Subanun of Mindanao' *American Anthropologist* 63: 113-32 (reprinted in Hymes, 1964).

Frake, C. O. (1962) 'The ethnographic study of cognitive systems' in T. Gladwin and W. Sturtevant (eds.) *Anthropology and Human Behavior*, Washington DC, Anthropological Society of Washington (reprinted in Tyler, 1969).

Freidson, E. (1971) *Profession of Medicine*, New York, Dodd, Mead.

Friedman, N. (1967) *The Social Nature of Psychological Research*, New York, Basic Books.

Garfinkel. H. (1964) 'Studies of the routine grounds of everyday activities' *Social Problems* 11: 225-50.

Garfinkel, H. (1967) *Studies in Ethnomethodology*, Englewood Cliffs, NJ, Prentice-Hall.

Giddens, A. (ed.) (1974) *Positivism and Sociology*, London, Heinemann.

Gilbert, B. B. (1966) *The Evolution of National Insurance in Great Britain: The Origins of the Welfare State*, London, Michael Joseph.

Goffman, E. (1968) *Asylums*, Harmondsworth, Penguin.

Goode, E. (1975) 'On behalf of labelling theory' *Social Problems* 22: 570-83.

Goodenough, W. H. (1964) 'Cultural anthropology and linguistics' in D. Hymes (ed.) *Language in Culture and Society*, New York, Harper and Row.

Goodenough W. H. (1965) 'Yankee kinship terminology: a problem in componential analysis' *American Anthropologist* 67: 259-87 (reprinted in Tyler, 1969).

Gould, H. (1957) 'The implications of technological change for folk and scientific medicine' *American Anthropologist* 59: 507-16.

Greene, R. (1971) *Sick Doctors*, London, Heinemann.

Habermas, J. (1971) *Toward a Rational Society*, London, Heinemann.

Harris, M. (1974) 'Why a perfect knowledge of all the rules one must know to act like a native cannot lead to the knowledge of how natives act' *Journal of Anthropological Research* 30: 242-51.

Horton, R. (1971) 'African traditional thought and western science' in M. F. D. Young (ed.) *Knowledge and Control*, London, Collier-Macmillan.

Hubert, J. (1974) 'Belief and reality: social factors in pregnancy and childbirth' in M. P. M. Richards (ed.) *The Integration of a Child into a Social World*, London, Cambridge University Press.

Hymes, D. (ed.) (1964) *Language in Culture and Society*, New York, Harper and Row.

Illich, I. (1975) *Medical Nemesis*, London, Calder and Boyars.

Kadushin, C. (1966) 'The friends and supporters of psychotherapy: on social circles in urban life' *American Sociological Review* 31: 786-802.

Keddie, N. (ed.) (1973) *Tinker, Tailor...The Myth of Cultural Deprivation* Harmondsworth, Penguin.

King, L. S. (1954) 'What is disease' *Philosophy of Science* 21: 193-203.

Kirscht, J. P., Haefner, D. P., Kegeles, S. S. and Rosenstock, I. M. (1966) 'A national study of health beliefs' *Journal of Health and Human Behavior* 7: 248-54.

Kosa, J., *et al.* (1966) 'The place of morbid episodes in the social interaction pattern' Paper presented to Sixth Congress of the International Sociological Association, Evian, France.

Kosa, J. and Robertson, L. S. (1969) 'The social aspects of health and illness' in J. Kosa, A. Antonovsky and I. K. Zola (eds.) *Poverty and Health*, Cambridge. MA., Harvard University Press.

Kuhn, T. S. (1970) *The Structure of Scientific Revolutions* (2nd edn.) Chicago, University of Chicago Press.

Landar, H. and Casagrande, J. (1962) 'Navaho anatomical reference' *Ethnology* 1: 370-3.

Lasch, C. (1975) 'What the doctor ordered' *New York Review of Books* 11 December.

Lefebvre, H. (1971) *Everyday Life in the Modern World*, London, Allen Lane.

Lemert, E. (1951) *Social Pathology*, New York, McGraw-Hill.

Lewis, A. (1953) 'Health as a social concept' *British Journal of Sociology* 4: 109-24.

Lewis, L. S. (1963) 'Rational behavior and the treatment of illness' *Journal of Health and Human Behavior* 4: 235-9.

Lewis, G. (1975) *Knowledge of Illness in a Sepik Society*, London, Athlone Press.

Lounsbury, F. G. (1964a) 'The structural analysis of kinship semantics' *Proceedings of the Ninth International Congress of Linguists* The Hague, Mouton (reprinted in Tyler, 1969).

Lounsbury, F. G. (1964b) 'A formal account of the Crow- and Omaha-type kinship terminologies' in W. H. Goodenough (ed..) *Explorations in Cultural Anthropology*, New York, McGraw-Hill (reprinted in Tyler, 1969).

MacAndrew, C. and Edgerton, R. B. (1970) *Drunken Comportment*, London, Nelson.

McHugh, P. (1970) 'A common-sense conception of deviance' in J. D. Douglas (ed.) *Deviance and Respectability*, New York, Basic Books.

McKinlay, J. B. (1972) 'Some approaches and problems in the study of the use of services - an overview' *Journal* of *Health and Social Behavior* 13: 115-52.

Manning, P. K. (1971) 'Fixing what you feared: notes on the campus abortion search' in J. M. Henslin (ed.) *Studies in the Sociology of Sex* New York, Appleton-Century-Crofts.

Marsh, G. H. and Laughlin, W. S. (1956) 'Human anatomical knowledge among the Aleutian Islanders' *Southwestern Journal of Anthropology* 12: 38-78.

Mechanic, D. (1962a) 'The concept of illness behavior' *Journal of Chronic Disease* 15: 189-94.

Mechanic, D. (1962b) *Students Under Stress: A Study of the Social Psychology of Adaptation*, New York, Free Press.

Mechanic, D. (1968) *Medical Sociology*, New York, Free Press.

Mechanic, D. and Volkart, E. H. (1961) 'Stress, illness behavior and the sick role' *American Sociological Review* 29: 51-8.

Metzger, D. and Williams, G. (1963) 'Tenejapa medicine I: the curer' *Southwestern Journal of Anthropology* 19: 217-34.

Moerman, M. (1974) 'Accomplishing ethnicity' in R. Turner (ed.) *Ethnomethodology*, Harmondsworth, Penguin.

Nagel, E. (1961) *The Structure of Science*, New York, Harcourt, Brace and World.

Parkin, F. (1967) 'Working class Conservatives', *British Journal of Sociology* 18: 278-90.

Parsons, T. (1951) *The Social System*, London, Routledge and Kegan Paul.

Parsons, T. and Fox, R. (1952) 'Illness, therapy and the modern American family' *Journal of Social Issues* 18: 31-44.

Phillips, D. L. (1972) 'Data collection as a social process: its implications for "true prevalence" studies of mental illness' in E. Freidson and J. Lorber (eds.) *Medical Men and Their Work*, Chicago, Aldine.

Phillips, D. L. (1973) *Abandoning Method*, London, Jossey-Bass.

Press, I. (1969) 'Urban illness: physicians, curers and dual use in Bogota' *Journal of Health and Social Behavior* 10: 209-18.

Psathas, G. (1968) 'Ethnomethods and phenomenology' *Social Research* 35: 501-20.

Puccetti, R. (1968) *Persons: A Study of Possible Moral Agents in the Universe*, London, Macmillan.

Rainwater, L. (1968) 'The lower class: health, illness and medical institutions' in I. Deutscher and E. Thompson (eds.) *Among the People*, New York, Basic Books.

Reif, L. (1973) Managing a life with chronic disease' *American Journal of Nursing* 73: 261-4.

Robinson, D. (1971) *The Process of Becoming Ill*, London, Routledge and Kegan Paul.

Rosenblatt, D. and Suchman, E. A. (1965) 'Blue-collar attitudes and information toward health and illness' in A. B. Shostak and W. Gomberg (eds.) *Blue-Collar World*, Englewood Cliffs, NJ, Prentice-Hall.

Rosenstock, I. M. (1966) 'Why people use health services' *Milbank Memorial Fund Quarterly* 64: 94-127.

Ross, E. A. (1901) *Social Control*, New York, Macmillan.

Rubel, A. J. (1960) 'Concepts of disease in Mexican-American culture' *American Anthropologist* 62: 795-814.

Rubel, A. J. (1964) 'The epidemiology of a folk illness: "Susto" in Hispanic America' *Ethnology* 3: 268-83.

Ryave, A. L. and Schenkein, J. N. (1974) 'Notes on the art of walking' in R. Turner (ed.) *Ethnomethodology*, Harmondsworth. Penguin.

Sacks, H. (1972) 'An initial investigation of the usability of conversational data for doing sociology' in D. Sudnow (ed.) *Studies in Social Interaction*, New York, Free Press.

Schroyer, T. (1971) 'The critical theory of late capitalism' in G. Fischer (ed.) *The Revival of American Socialism*, New York, Oxford University Press.

Schulman, S. and Smith, A. M. (1963) 'The concept of "health" among Spanish-speaking villagers of New Mexico and Colorado' *Journal of Health and Human Behavior* 4: 226-34.

Schutz, A. (1962) *Collected Papers Vol. 1: The Problem of Social Reality*, The Hague, Martinus Nijhoff.

Schutz, A. (1964) *Collected Papers Vol. II: Studies in Social Theory*, The Hague, Martinus Nijhoff.

Schutz, A. (1970) *Reflections on the Problems of Relevance*, New Haven, Yale University Press.

Schutz, A. and Luckmann, T. (1974) *The Structures of the Life-World*, London, Heinemann.

Schwartz, L. R. (1969) 'The hierarchy of resort in curative practices: The Admiralty Islands, Melanesia' *Journal of Health and Social Behavior* 20: 1-9.

Scott, M. B. (1968) *The Racing Game*, Chicago, Aldine.

Sedgwick, P. (1972) 'Mental Illness *is* Illness' Paper presented to the National Deviancy Conference, Tenth Deviancy Symposium, York. [Published as part of Chapter 1 in P. Sedgwick, *Psychopolitics*, London, Pluto Press, 1982].

Stark, L. R. (1969) 'The lexical structure of Quechua body parts' *Anthropological Linguistics* 2: 1-15.

Strauss, A. L. (1969) 'Medical organisation, medical care and lower income groups' *Social Science and Medicine* 3: 143-77.

Suchman, E. A. (1964) 'Sociomedical variations among ethnic groups' *American Journal of Sociology* 70: 319-31.

Suchman, E. A. (1965) 'Stages of illness and medical care' *Journal of Health and Human Behavior* 6: 114-28.

Sudnow, D. (1967) *Passing On: The Social Organisation of Dying*, Englewood Cliffs, NJ, Prentice-Hall.

Sudnow, D. (ed.) (1972) *Studies in Social Interaction*, New York, Free Press.

Thompson, B. (1967) 'Childbirth and infant care in a West African village' *Nursing Mirror* 29 September.

Thompson, B. and Baird, D. (1967a) 'Some impressions of childbearing in tropical areas: Part I' *The Journal of Obstetrics and Gynaecology of the British Commonwealth* 74; 329-38.

Thompson, B. and Baird, D. (1967b) 'Some impressions of childbearing in tropical areas: Parts II and III' *The Journal of Obstetrics and Gynaecology of the British Commonwealth* 74: 499-522.

Turner, R. (ed.) (1974) *Ethnomethodology*, Harmondsworth, Penguin.

Twaddle, A. C. (1973) 'Illness and deviance' *Social Science and Medicine* 7: 751-62.

Tyler, S. A. (1969) *Cognitive Anthropology*, New York, Holt, Rhinehart, Winston.

Voysey, M. (1975) *A Constant Burden*, London, Routledge and Kegan Paul.

Waddington, I. (1973) 'The role of the hospital in the development of modern medicine: a sociological analysis' *Sociology* 7: 211-24.

Wallace, A. F. C. and Atkins, J. (1960) 'The meaning of kinship terms' *American Anthropologist* 62: 58-80 (reprinted in Tyler, 1969).

Warren, C. A. B. (1974) *Identity and Community in the Gay World*, New York, Wiley.

Warren, C. A. B. and Johnson, J. M. (1972) 'A critique of labelling theory from the phenomenological perspective' in R. A. Scott and J. D. Douglas (eds.) *Theoretical Perspectives on Deviance*, New York, Basic Books.

Watson, W. (1964) 'Social mobility and social class in industrial communities' in M. Gluckman (ed.) *Closed Systems and Open Minds*, Chicago, Aldine.

Weinberg, M. S. (1970) 'The nudist management of respectability: strategy for, and consequences of, the construction of a situated morality' in J. D. Douglas (ed.) *Deviance and Respectability*, New York, Basic Books.

Wieder, D. L. (1974) 'On meaning by rule' in J. D. Douglas (ed.) *Understanding Everyday Life*, London, Routledge and Kegan Paul.

Wittgenstein, L. (1972) *Philosophical Investigations*, Oxford, Blackwell.

Wittgenstein, L. (1974) *Tractatus Logico-Philosophicus*, London, Routledge and Kegan Paul.

Wolff, M. (1973) 'Notes on the behaviour of pedestrians' in A. Birenbaum and E. Sagarin (eds.) *People in Places*, London, Nelson.

Wootton, A. (1975) *Dilemmas of Discourse*, London, Allen and Unwin.

Young, J. (1971) *The Drugtakers*, London, Paladin.

Zborowski, M. (1952) 'Cultural components in responses to pain' *Journal of Social Issues* 8: 16-30.

Zimmerman, D. H. and Wieder, D. L. (1971) 'Ethnomethodology and the problem of order: comment on Denzin' in J. D. Douglas (ed.) *Understanding Everyday Life*, London, Routledge and Kegan Paul.

Zola, I. K. (1965) 'Illness behavior of the working class' in A. B. Shostak and W. Gomberg (eds.) *Blue-Collar World*, Englewood Cliffs, NJ, Prentice-Hall.

Zola, I. K. (1966) 'Culture and symptoms: an analysis of patients' presenting complaints' *American Sociological Review* 31: 615-30.

Additional References to the 2001 Edition

Abbott, A. (1988) *The System of Professions*, Chicago, University of Chicago Press.

Abbott, A. (2001) *Chaos of Disciplines*, Chicago, University of Chicago Press.

Agar, M. H. (1973) *Ripping and running : a formal ethnography of urban heroin addicts*, London, Seminar Press.

Agar, M. H. (1980) *The Professional Stranger: An Informal Introduction to Ethnography*, London, Academic Press.

Agar, M. H. (1996) *The Professional Stranger: An Informal Introduction to Ethnography*, (Second Edition) San Diego: Academic Press.

Agar, M. (1982) 'Whatever happened to cognitive anthropology - a partial review *Human Organization* 41: 82-6.

Becker, M. H., Drachman, R. H. and Kirscht, J. P. 'Motivations as predictors of health behavior' *Health Services Report* 87: 852.

Camic, C. (1987) 'The making of a method: a historical reinterpretation of the early Parsons' *American Sociological Review* 52:421-439.

Conner, M. and Norman, P., eds. (1996) *Predicting Health Behaviour; Research and Practice with Social Cognition Models*, Buckingham, Open University Press.

De Mille, R. (1976) *Castaneda's Journey: The Power and the Allegory*, Santa Barbara, Capra.

De Mille, R., ed. (1980) *The Don Juan Papers: Further Castaneda Controversies*, Santa Barbara, Ross-Erikson.

Dingwall, R. (1997) 'Accounts, interviews and observation' pp.51-65 in Miller, G. and Dingwall, R., eds., *Context and Method in Qualitative Research*, London, Sage.

Freidson, E. (1986) *Professional Powers: A Study of the Institutionalization of Formal Knowledge*, Chicago, University of Chicago Press.

Freidson, E. (1994) *Professionalism Reborn: Theory, Prophecy and Policy*, Cambridge, Polity Press.

Goffman, E. (1983) 'Felicity's Condition' *American Journal of Sociology* 89; 1:1-53.

Hughes, E. (1971) *The Sociological Eye: Selected Papers on Work, Self and the Study of Society*, Chicago, Aldine-Atherton.

Hutchins, E. (1980) *Culture and Inference*, Cambridge, Harvard University Press.

Rosenstock, I.M., Strecher, V.J. and Becker, M.H. (1988) ' Social learning theory and the health belief model' *Health Education Quarterly* 15: 175-183.

Sacks, H., Schegloff, E. A. and Jefferson, G. (1974) 'A simplest systematics for the organization of turn-taking for conversation' *Language* 50: 696-735.

Sacks, H. (1995) *Lectures on Conversation*, Oxford, Blackwell.

Sarat, A. and Silbey, S. (1988) 'The pull of the policy audience' *Law and Policy* 10; 2/3: 97-166.

Spradley, J. (1979) *The Ethnographic Interview*, Fort Worth, Harcourt Brace Jovanovich.

Subject Index

Author Index